EMERGENCY AND INTENSIVE CARE MEDICINE

AF734567

APPENDICITIS

PREVALENCE, RISK FACTORS AND CLINICAL MANAGEMENT

Emergency and Intensive Care Medicine

Additional books and e-books in this series can be found on Nova's website under the Series tab.

Digestive Diseases – Research and Clinical Developments

Additional books and e-books in this series can be found on Nova's website under the Series tab.

EMERGENCY AND INTENSIVE CARE MEDICINE

APPENDICITIS

PREVALENCE, RISK FACTORS AND CLINICAL MANAGEMENT

ROSE BALLARD
EDITOR

nova
Medicine & Health
New York

Library of Congress Cataloging-in-Publication Data

ISBN: 978-1-53614-753-7

Published by Nova Science Publishers, Inc. † New York

CONTENTS

PREFACE

Acute appendicitis is one of the most common surgical abdominal emergencies worldwide, with a lifetime risk of 8.6% for males and 6.7% for females. This compilation discusses how while non-operative treatment of appendicitis has been proposed as an alternative to surgery, appendicectomy remains the mainstay of treatment in most cases and techniques have shifted from open to laparoscopic methods. The current knowledge in pathogenesis, diagnosis, and clinical management of acute appendicitis is also discussed.

Next, the authors present an updated review chapter of appendicitis regarding its prevalence and risk factors, particularly how the diagnosis of appendicitis is based on a history of diffuse abdominal pain, which usually starts in the central region of the abdomen and migrates to the lower right quadrant of the abdomen.

The residual remnant or "stump" of the appendix after an initial appendectomy may become inflamed causing what is commonly referred to as stump appendicitis. Treatment with antibiotics may be attempted as an alternative to surgery; however, the vast majority of cases require definitive surgical excision of the remnant appendix. The authors propose that keeping this disease in the differential is important in reducing complications associated with delayed diagnosis.

Chapter 1 - Acute appendicitis is one of the commonest surgical abdominal emergencies worldwide, with a lifetime risk of 8.6% for males and 6.7% for females. Yet, the aetiology remains uncertain and diagnosis is largely based on clinical judgement. Biomarkers and imaging are useful to support the diagnosis, but cannot be utilised in isolation, as they may be misleading. Clinical scoring systems have a high negative predictive value but are less reliable rule-in tools. With the prevalent age group being the second decade of life, the clinical picture can vary from subtle signs and symptoms to life-threatening sepsis. Clinical classification creates a necessary divide in management between simple and complex appendicitis. Whilst non-operative treatment of appendicitis has been proposed as an alternative to surgery, appendicectomy remains the mainstay of treatment in most cases and techniques have shifted from open to laparoscopic methods. Mortality rate is low, but post-operative complications are common in complex disease. The authors discuss the current knowledge in pathogenesis, diagnosis, and clinical management of acute appendicitis.

Chapter 2 - *Background:* Acute appendicitis affects an average of 70,000 American children a year, being the main cause of abdominal surgeries in children. The appendix can be found perforated in up to one third of appendectomies. The diagnosis of appendicitis is based on a history of diffuse abdominal pain, which usually starts in the central region of the abdomen and migrates to the lower right quadrant of the abdomen. It can vary on its clinical presentation due to the anatomical variation of the vermiform appendix. Appendectomy is still the standard treatment for acute appendicitis but clinical management should be considered in some specific situations.

Aim: The aim of this chapter is to present an updated review chapter of appendicitis regarding its prevalence, risk factors and clinical management.

Method: The chapter was written based on recent articles found on online scientific databases using the keywords: Appendicitis; Prevalence; Risk Factors; Clinical management.

Conclusion: Acute appendicitis is the most common surgical acute disease of the abdominal and has always to be considered in a young patient with abdominal pain. Patients diagnosed with local abscess may require previous clinical treatment before surgery and can be conducted with venous antibiotic therapy and elective appendectomy. Early surgical treatment when appendicitis is complicated with local abscess is associated with higher morbidity compared to initial conservative treatment. Cases of clinical management are exception and all the patients have to be exanimated by a surgeon.

Chapter 3 - The residual remnant or "stump" of the appendix after an initial appendectomy may become inflamed causing what is commonly referred to as stump appendicitis. The incidence of stump appendicitis is estimated to be 1 in 50,000 cases, making the diagnosis exceedingly rare. This uncommon disease coupled with a prior history of appendectomy can lead to a delay in diagnosis. While no single cause has been identified, there is evidence to suggest that the length of the residual stump after resection has an influence on recurrent infection. The difficulty in the diagnosis of the disease lies in its ambiguous presentation in the setting of a presumed completely resected appendix. Unfortunately, giving the often nonspecific vital signs and inconclusive laboratory results as the initial available data, a physician will need to maintain a high clinical suspicion in order to make the correct diagnosis. The use of computed tomography (CT) scans has reduced the need for more invasive diagnostic techniques and aids in the physician's ability to expeditiously diagnose stump appendicitis. Ultrasonography has also been demonstrated to aid in the diagnosis of stump appendicitis, particularly where CT scans are not as readily available. Treatment with antibiotics may be attempted as an alternative to surgery; however, the vast majority of cases require definitive surgical excision of the remnant appendix. Stump appendicitis is a problematic disease with an underestimated prevalence. Delays in diagnosis can lead to significant patient morbidity and more complex surgical procedures. Keeping this disease in the differential is important in reducing complications associated with delayed diagnosis.

In: Appendicitis
Editor: Rose Ballard

ISBN: 978-1-53614-753-7

Chapter 1

APPENDICITIS: CURRENT KNOWLEDGE, TRENDS AND PRACTICE

Neville Spiteri* and Paul Skaife
Department of Colorectal Surgery, Aintree University Hospital, Liverpool, UK

ABSTRACT

Acute appendicitis is one of the commonest surgical abdominal emergencies worldwide, with a lifetime risk of 8.6% for males and 6.7% for females. Yet, the aetiology remains uncertain and diagnosis is largely based on clinical judgement. Biomarkers and imaging are useful to support the diagnosis, but cannot be utilised in isolation, as they may be misleading. Clinical scoring systems have a high negative predictive value but are less reliable rule-in tools. With the prevalent age group being the second decade of life, the clinical picture can vary from subtle signs and symptoms to life-threatening sepsis. Clinical classification creates a necessary divide in management between simple and complex appendicitis. Whilst non-operative treatment of appendicitis has been proposed as an alternative to surgery, appendicectomy remains the mainstay of treatment in most cases and techniques have shifted from open to laparoscopic methods. Mortality rate is low, but post-operative

* Corresponding Author Email: neville.spiteri@gov.mt.

complications are common in complex disease. We discuss the current knowledge in pathogenesis, diagnosis, and clinical management of acute appendicitis.

Keywords: appendix, appendicitis

Introduction

Acute appendicitis has withstood the test of time as one of the commonest surgical emergencies requiring operative intervention. With a lifetime risk of 8.6% for males and 6.7% for females [1], it is a frequent culprit for cases of acute abdominal pain presenting to the emergency department, and can lead to significant morbidity, and even mortality. Symptoms and signs are very often non-specific, however, and acute appendicitis is invariably listed in the differential diagnosis of most, if not all, cases presenting with acute abdominal pain.

Despite being so common, aetiology is still poorly understood, diagnostic tools remain unreliable and best practice guidance varies between care-givers internationally. This leads to variations in hospital stay, timing of surgery – if at all – and general outcomes.

Physiological Role of the Appendix

The appendix is a lymphoid organ, with a role in B-lymphocyte-mediated immune response and extra-thymically derived T-lymphocytes [2].

It might also act as a reservoir for gut microbes, becoming important when gut flora are diminished, for example [3]. This might explain, in part, the increased risk of severe *Clostridium difficile* colitis in appendicectomy patients [4].

The mechanism is unclear, but the reduced risk of developing ulcerative colitis in patients who had their appendix removed [5], and the increased risk of developing Crohn's disease [6] might be related to the organ's functions.

Epidemiology of Appendicitis

Acute appendicitis is a worldwide disease, albeit incidence bears geographical variation. Dr. Reginald Heber Fitz was the first to describe appendicitis in 1886 [7]. Since then, the incidence has risen, fallen, and then plateaued in Western countries. Newly industrialised countries appear to be only in the first stage of this sequence [8].

The incidence of appendicitis in the 21st century was quantified to be around 100 per 100,000 inhabitants in Northern America, 105 in Eastern Europe and 151 in Western Europe [8].

White individuals seem to have a higher propensity for appendicitis, according to population-based studies [9], although the reason is unclear.

Incidence of appendicitis seems to peak in persons in their second decade of life (23.3 per 10,000 population per year) [1], with males having slightly higher rates of appendicitis (male to female ratio of 1.4:1 in one study [1]), despite lifetime appendicectomy rates being lower than those for females (12% versus 24%) [10], probably due to gynaecological pathology mimicking appendicitis.

Pregnancy seems to be protective for appendicitis, especially around the third trimester [11].

Aetiology and Risk Factors of Appendicitis

Aetiology of appendicitis remains uncertain, but there are several postulated causes [3, 12].

Luminal obstruction with subsequent increase in intra-luminal pressure due to build-up of mucosal secretions may lead to vascular compromise, with engorgement leading to necrosis and perforation. The obstruction may be secondary to a faecolith, lymphoid hyperplasia, impacted stool or tumour [13].

Genetic predisposition was hypothesised to play a part in twin studies and patients with positive family history [14, 15], with the risk being three-fold in patients with a positive family history.

Microbial triggers have been documented [16], but are not directly linked to development of appendicitis.

Seasonal variation in presentation, with a predominance of incidence in the summer months, has been documented [17] – although this might be linked to pollution levels rather than nature itself.

Proliferation of appendicular nerve fibres, with subsequent increase in neuropeptides, leading to appendix-related pain, in a macroscopically normal appendix might explain the improvement in pain after a normal appendicectomy. This, so-called neurogenic appendicitis has been described as a common diagnosis in children [18].

It is probable that multiple of the aforementioned factors come into play, with the scales tipping towards inflammation when there is enough causation to do so.

Clinical Features of Appendicitis

Acute appendicitis can produce a multitude of signs and symptoms, often related to patient factors, the timing of presentation following onset, its lie, and the severity of appendicitis.

The classical history is that of central (mid-gut) abdominal pain, which over a period of 12-24 hours localises to the right iliac fossa, due to peritoneal irritation. This migratory pain has been shown in a meta-analysis to be the strongest symptom linked with a diagnosis of acute appendicitis [19]. There may be associated gastro-intestinal symptoms such as nausea, vomiting or diarrhoea. Clinical examination often yields the findings of a pyrexial patient, with evolving right iliac fossa peritonism.

In the absence of peritoneal irritation, the likelihood ratio of acute appendicitis was only 0.24 - 0.39 in a meta-analysis [19], with the psoas and Rovsing's signs being of limited diagnostic value.

Investigations

The history and clinical examination are sometimes sufficient to confirm the diagnosis of appendicitis, however it is often the case that further information is required to exclude other causes, but also to stratify appendicitis into simple or complex, as will be discussed later in this chapter.

Biomarkers

Whilst blood investigations are often obtained as a routine baseline, to exclude other causes, and to assess parameters such as kidney function, no isolated biomarker is sufficiently specific for appendicitis [20]. Nonetheless, a rise in inflammatory markers such as white cell count, granulocyte count, polymorphonuclear cell percentage and/or C-reactive protein (CRP) makes appendicitis more likely [19] (*Table 1*).

Table 1. Predictive power of biomarkers in appendicitis

Biomarker	Value	LR	P Value
White Cell Count	$\geq 10x10^9/l$	2.47	< 0.001
Granulocyte Count	$\geq 7x10^9/l$	1.64	< 0.001
Polymorphonuclear Cell Percentage	> 75%	2.44	0.001
CRP	> 10mg/l	1.97	< 0.001

Adapted from: REB Andersson, Meta-analysis of the clinical and laboratory diagnosis of appendicitis, BJS 2004; 91: 28-37

A number of new inflammatory markers (interleukin-6, chemokine ligand-8, chemokine C-C motif ligand-2, serum amyloid A, matrix metalloproteinase-9 and myeloperoxidase) have been identified in the literature as promising, but none have been shown to be sufficiently sensitive for use in clinical practice [21]. Procalcitonin may have a role in identifying complicated appendicitis [20].

Urinalysis

The inflamed appendix may lie near the ureter and patients may have blood or leucocytes in their urine, hence whilst urinalysis may supplement a differential diagnosis of a urinary tract infection, one must keep this in mind.

In women of child-bearing age, it is important to obtain a urine pregnancy test to rule out pregnancy as a cause of symptoms, but also to safeguard the foetus in cases of appendicitis in pregnancy.

Clinical Scoring Systems

Multifactorial scoring systems based on clinical and biochemical information are often easy to use and reproducible. The most popular of these are the Alvarado (also known as the MANTRELS) score and the Appendicitis Inflammatory Response (AIR) score. The Paediatric Appendicitis Score (PAS), the Raja Isteri Pengiran Anak Saleha Appendicitis (RIPASA) score and the Adult Appendicitis Score (AAS) are also well documented in the literature. The World Society of Emergency Surgery (WSES) compare these scores in their guidelines for diagnosis and treatment of appendicitis [22].

Whilst most of these scores' data are based on data from level 2 and 3 evidence, the Alvarado score has been extensively studied and validated. The 10-point score is based on 3 clinical symptoms (abdominal pain migrating to the right iliac fossa, anorexia, nausea or vomiting), 3 clinical signs (right iliac fossa tenderness, pyrexia and rebound tenderness) and 2 biochemical values (leucocytosis and left white cell count shift). In a systematic review by Ohle et al. [23] that included 5960 patients in 29 studies, a cut-off value of less than ruled out acute appendicitis with a sensitivity of 99% (95% Confidence Interval (CI): 97 - 99%), but a specificity of only 43% (CI: 36 - 51%). The score over-predicted the probability of appendicitis in females and performed inconsistently in the paediatric population but was well-calibrated in males.

The AIR Score, published in 2008 [24], is based on clinical signs and symptoms (vomiting, right iliac fossa pain, rebound tenderness, pyrexia, polymorphonuclear leukocytes, leukocystosis) and a raised CRP. The score performed better than the Alvarado score for diagnosis of acute appendicitis, with receiver-operator curve (ROC) area of 0.97 for advanced appendicitis, versus the 0.92 of the Alvarado score ($p = 0.0027$) and 0.93 versus 0.88 for all appendicitis, respectively (p = 0.0007). The AIR score was externally validated by de Castro et al. [25] and can act as a guide in decision-making to reduce hospital stay, admissions, further investigation and negative exploration [26, 27] (Table 2).

Being common in the paediatric population, acute appendicitis often poses a more difficult challenge to diagnose than in the adult population. The history is a challenge to obtain and frequently depends on the child's vocabulary, observation is sometimes logistically difficult, and imaging is most often reserved for the most challenging of cases and negative exploration can carry morbidity. Hence, standardisation of clinical findings and devising a clinical score is not easy. The Paediatric Appendicitis Score (PAS) [28] was published in 2002, based on a population of 1,170 children. 8 variables are taken into account: cough/percussion tenderness in the right iliac fossa, anorexia, pyrexia, nausea/vomiting, right iliac fossa tenderness, leucocytosis, polymorphonuclear neutrophilia and migration of pain to the right iliac fossa. It had a positive predictive value of 0.96 and a negative predictive value of 0.99 in this population. This score was compared to the Alvarado score in a systematic review [29] and the latter outperformed the PAS.

Table 2. AIR score risk stratification and proposed clinical management

Score	Risk	Recommendation
0-4	Low	Outpatient follow up
5-8	Intermediate	Inpatient observation or further investigation
9-12	High	Surgical exploration

Most of these studies, and other literature comparing or validating these and similar scores are based on a cohort of patients who, in the majority, have undergone appendicectomy. This leads to a potential skewing of results. Additionally, there are basic demographic differences and heterogeneity in investigative modalities and treatment options between countries. One therefore questions the reproducibility of such scores on the general population presenting at the (local) accident and emergency department.

The WSES guidelines suggest that the Alvarado score is sufficiently sensitive to exclude acute appendicitis at a cut-off of < 5, but none of the scores published is sufficiently sensitive and specific to be clinically useful in confirming the disease [22]. Clinical judgement, therefore, remains the most important factor in diagnosis of acute appendicitis.

Imaging

Whilst plain x-rays are still useful to reject other pathologies in the list of differential diagnoses, modalities that have been evaluated in the management of acute appendicitis include ultrasonography (US), computed tomography (CT) and magnetic resonance imaging (MRI).

The diagnosis of acute appendicitis, can sometimes be challenging and clinical assessment alone does not suffice. Patient groups such as pregnant women, women of child-bearing age and the elderly may pose diagnostic dilemmas. The middle-aged patient who presents with atypical – or even typical – symptoms is a concern, given that appendicitis is less frequent in this age-group, diverticulosis is common, and malignancy forms part of the differential diagnosis.

CT is the most utilised imaging modality in the adult population, and in a Washington-based study, 86% of adult patients who underwent an appendicectomy had a prior CT scan [30], with a sensitivity of 92.3% and a negative appendicectomy rate of 6%.

The clinical scenario where simple acute appendicitis is much more likely than any other diagnosis is common, and in this situation, imaging seldom proves useful. Exposing such patients to further investigation is often not required and raises concerns about risks of unnecessary radiation exposure and utilisation of resources. Arguments in favour of this approach include the fact that laparoscopy is a highly sensitive and relatively safe procedure [31]. In contrast, it is common for imaging to form part of the primary assessment of the same presenting complaint in geographical areas where access to scans is easy and medicolegal pressure high, with the benefit of reduction in normal appendectomy rates. Furthermore, there is increasing evidence that spontaneous resolution of acute appendicitis is common and that imaging can improve detection of such benign forms [32].

Ultrasonography is a safe modality, which can alleviate concerns about radiation exposure. It is, however, operator-dependent and often unavailable out-of-hours. Sensitivity was 86% (95% CI: 83-88%), and specificity was 81% (CI 78-84) in a systematic review [33], hence leading to concerns about false negative results.

MRI, like US, eliminates the risks associated with radiation exposure. It is however a limited resource which is scantily available in the acute setting and, subsequently, there is little literature documenting its utility in acute appendicitis With sensitivity and specificity comparable to US (supplemented by selective CT) [34], there is currently not enough evidence to justify its use in everyday practice. One exception might be the pregnant patient with an equivocal clinical diagnosis, despite US evaluation. In such scenarios, MRI has been shown to have a lower non-visualisation rate than ultrasound [35].

Atema et al. [36] described a scoring system that combined clinical and radiological features to distinguish uncomplicated from complicated appendicitis, with 95% of patients deemed to have uncomplicated appendicitis being correctly identified as such.

There is no scoring system for diagnosis of acute appendicitis that combines clinical and radiological parameters; and the clinical picture of this condition is as heterogenous as the infrastructures of hospitals around the world. It, therefore, very often falls to the surgical team to make use of the available resources and stratify the patients accordingly. Clinical and biochemical information is key to estimating likelihood of acute appendicitis and tailoring management accordingly. The Alvarado or AIR Scores are the currently available stratification tools that can aid clinical decision-making and requests for imaging. Whereas low-risk patients can be managed in an ambulatory setting, high-risk patients require admission and will, in all likelihood, require surgery, with or without preceding imaging – depending on local resources and guidelines. Intermediate-risk patients are those who will benefit most from observation and/or imaging, with CT being performed primarily or following a negative US (if still clinically indicated), depending on local guidelines (Figure 1).

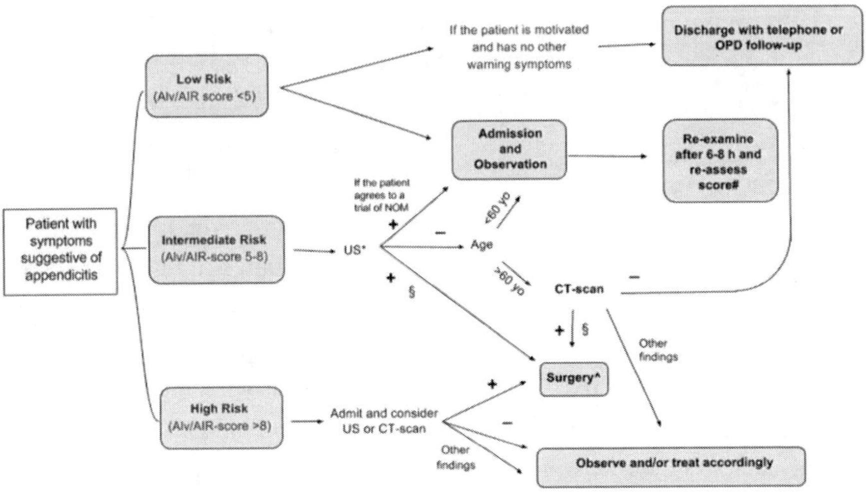

* If possible US Standard reporting templates for ultrasound and US 3 step sequential positioning; consider routine use of CT scan upon setting (e.g., USA) for Intermediate risk group; consider further imaging (US or CT) by carefully weighting risks/benefits of radiation exposure in low risk group

\# If no improvements after observation and re-assessment. Consider CT scan

§ Consider NOM + antibiotics in patients with severe comorbidities and high anesthesilogical risk

^ Surgery is meant as Acute Appendectomy. In case of finding of abscess or phlegmon on US/CT, consider percutaneous drainage if interventional radiology is available.

Reproduced from Di Saverio et al. World Journal of Emergency Surgery (2016) 11:34.

Figure 1. Practical WSES algorithm for diagnosis and treatment of patients with suspected acute appendicitis.

Classification of Acute Appendicitis

Acute appendicitis is classified by the European Association of Endoscopic Surgery (EAES) into simple (or uncomplicated) appendicitis –

without gangrene or necrosis, that does not progress to perforation – and complicated appendicitis, which results in a gangrenous appendix with or without perforation, peri-appendicular contained abscess or intra-abdominal abscess [37]. Classification has evolved with treatment strategies, and the WSES further subdivide simple appendicitis into normal-looking or inflamed, and complicated appendicitis into necrotic, inflammatory or perforated [38] (Table 3).

Table 3. WSES proposed grading system of acute appendicitis based on clinical, imaging and laparoscopic findings

Type	Grade	Description
Non-Complicated	0 – Normal	Normal looking appendix
	1 – Inflamed	Hyperemia, oedema +/- fibrin without or little pericolic fluid
Complicated	2 – Necrotic	A – Segmental necrosis B – Necrosis of base
	3 – Inflammatory	A – Phlegmon B – Abscess <5cm without free air C – Abscess >5cm without free air
	4 – Perforated	Diffuse peritonitis with or without free air

Reproduced from Gomes et al. World Journal of Emergency Surgery (2015) 10:60.

Classification is necessary as treatment strategies may differ; and there is probably a pathophysiological reason for this difference. In 2007, Livingston et al. [39] published a population-based observational study on secular trends in appendicitis and appendicectomy rates in the United States. They noted a decline in non-perforated appendicitis but not in perforated appendicitis, despite an increase in appendicectomies and more frequent use of CT imaging and laparoscopy. There was also no relationship between negative appendicectomy and perforation rates. They suggest that this disconnection of trends might be due to different pathophysiology between perforated and non-perforated appendicitis and hence that non-operative management may have a role in the initial management of non-perforating appendicitis. This was further reinforced by Ruber et al. [40], who – in 2010 – found that there was a difference in the pattern of circulating inflammatory markers between patients with gangrenous and phlegmonous appendicitis.

They suggest that the two are different entities with divergent immune regulation.

MANAGEMENT OF ACUTE APPENDICITIS

Treatment strategies will bear some geographical differences, and our aim here is to discuss current knowledge about the available treatment options.

Non-Operative Approach

We have already discussed the probability that simple appendicitis is pathophysiologically different from complicated appendicitis. It follows, therefore, that there may be a role for non-operative treatment for this cohort of patients. Several studies have evaluated this possibility.

In 2010, Varadhan et al. [41] published a meta-analysis, comparing 470 patients treated with antibiotics with 430 patients treated with appendicectomy. After 1 year, 63% of the patients did not require an operation or further treatment. Relative risk reduction was of 31%. There were no significant differences for length of stay or risk of developing complicated appendicitis.

The Non-Operative Treatment for Acute Appendicitis (NOTA) study [42] was a prospective study whereby 159 patients with suspected appendicitis, were treated with antibiotics (amoxicillin/clauvanate) and followed up for 2 years. 2-year efficacy of non-operative management was 83% (118 patients' recurrence free). There was a 13.8% (n = 22) 1-year recurrence rate – albeit 14 patients from the 22 were then successfully treated conservatively. Mean length of stay for the patients was 0.4 days.

Svensson et al. [43] published a randomised controlled trial in 2015, evaluating conservative management in young patients. 50 paediatric patients were randomised to antibiotic treatment (n = 24) or appendicectomy (n = 26). 92% of the antibiotic arm had initial resolution of symptoms, with

38% of the patients in the same arm eventually undergoing appendicectomy - 1 patient had proven acute appendicitis, but 6 had recurrent abdominal pain but non-conclusive histology.

The APPAC (Antibiotic Treatment versus Appendicectomy for Treatment of Uncomplicated Acute Appendicitis) trial [44] randomised 530 CT-confirmed, uncomplicated appendicitis into those treated with antibiotics (n = 257) and those treated with appendicectomy (n = 273). There was a 27% 1-year recurrence and appendicectomy rate in the antibiotic group.

These studies do, however, have some limitations, including different diagnostic criteria, use of imaging to confirm diagnosis in patients treated conservatively, low inclusion rate of eligible patients, and differences in follow up.

Moreover, the perceived role of antibiotics in the treatment of this cohort of patients may be creating bias, as some of these cases might be resolving spontaneously.

In summary, antibiotic therapy may be useful in patients with simple appendicitis who do not want surgery, accepting the risk of around 30% failure of conservative management. The question arises as to the duration of antibiotic treatment in this cohort of patients.

One must keep in mind the possibility of malignancy, especially in patients over 40 years of age. It would be wise to refer such patients for colonoscopy.

Operative Approach

Appendicectomy technique has evolved substantially since Claudius Amyand utilised a scrotal incision to resect the appendix lying in an inguinoscrotal hernia of an 11-year old boy.

Open and laparoscopic techniques are both widely advocated. The latter has gained popularity as the approach of choice where the equipment and expertise is available. This is mainly due to the advantages of decreased pain and subsequent decreased length of stay and earlier return to work [45, 46].

Similarly, a shorter length of stay has also been demonstrated in the paediatric population [47], albeit with morbidity comparable to the open approach.

It is an especially useful diagnostic tool in women of childbearing age, in whom there is overlap of symptoms between ovarian and appendiceal pathologies. There is currently no strong evidence to favour laparoscopic over open appendicectomy in the pregnant population. There might, in fact, be a higher rate of foetal loss with the laparoscopic approach [48]. We will discuss the management of this cohort of patients later in this chapter.

The laparoscopic approach was associated with a shorter length of stay and improved clinical outcomes for patients older than 65 years, with co-morbidities, and with complicated appendicitis in two large population based studies [49, 50].

Laparoscopic appendicectomy has a documented longer operative time (albeit of only up to 18.3 minutes) with the laparoscopic approach, and there seems to be a higher rate of intra-abdominal infection in both the adult [51, 52] and paediatric population [47].

The open approach to appendicectomy maintains a role where equipment or expertise is not available, as well as cases where laparoscopy is contra-indicated. The scenario where a laparoscopic procedure is converted to open is rare nowadays due to improved expertise and equipment, but in cases where this is necessary – similar to most difficult laparoscopic cases for other pathologies – experience and knowledge of the open technique is of the essence.

Common Themes on Operative Technique

- Port placement depends on surgeon preference and experience. The authors prefer a 10-12mm infra-umbilical camera port, established in a modified Hasson approach whenever possible, along with 5mm left iliac fossa and suprapubic ports, both inserted under vision. When inserting the latter, care should be taken to avoid the urinary bladder and one will find that diverting just lateral to the urachus on insertion avoids this embarrassment.

- It is wise to perform a laparoscopy at the start of the procedure. This helps with differential diagnoses such as Meckel's diverticulum, identifies any distant pockets of pus and avoids forgetting to do it at the end of the procedure.
- The appendix mesentery should be taken with the specimen and not left behind due to the risk of appendiceal carcinoid mesenteric involvement.
- The use of diathermy to dissect the mesoappendix increases the risk of bleeding and thermal injury but remains the most cost-effective option compared to the described use of endoclips, stapling devices, ligasure and harmonic scalpel, and is safe in experienced hands. An elegant technique described by Motson et al. [53] involves the creation of a mesenteric window at the level of the appendix base, division of the appendix at this point with scissors and securing the appendix stump and mesentery with consecutive endoloops.
- There is no advantage of stump inversion over simple ligation and the latter is advocated to be simpler and faster, whilst preserving caecal wall anatomy [54, 55].
- Lavage of the peritoneum does not offer any advantage over simple suctioning of any pus on its own [56].
- The employment of drains is a contentious issue, mainly due to the belief that they may reduce abscess formation, but literature has failed to prove the advantage of their use and suggests that they may cause an increased operative time, length of stay and incidence of wound infection [57, 58].

Note should be made that there are other approaches to appendicectomy and these include single-incision laparoscopic surgery (SILS) and natural orifice transluminal endoscopic surgery (NOTES). These techniques have not – to date – gained widespread adoption due to their higher cost and increased complexity with no marked advantages [59]–[61].

SPECIFIC TOPICS AND DECISION-MAKING

Timing of Surgery

The probability that uncomplicated – hence, non-perforating – and complicated – hence perforating – appendicitis are separate entities, and therefore have different natural histories, suggests that timing of intervention is not critical in all cases of appendicitis. The septic patient requires urgent surgery. On the other hand, observation of patients who are not unwell is an excellent strategy, and it will filter out patients who do not have appendicitis or resolve spontaneously, whilst increasing diagnostic accuracy. Perforation rate is a misleading indicator in this instance, since conservative management of some patients can increase the proportion of perforated appendicitis in those who are operated, but the number of perforations stays the same. Short delays of 24 hours [62], but not more than 72 hours [63], in patients who are not septic, should ensure no increase in the rate of complex appendicitis. Such delays may aid hospital service provision, avoiding night-time operations, whilst prioritising patients for surgery.

It is therefore reasonable to plan surgery for uncomplicated appendicitis for the next available emergency list.

The Normal Appendix

There is variation in practice in cases where a normal appendix is found in a symptomatic patient with no other explanatory pathology. There is evidence to show that a macroscopically normal appendix may still be pathological and, subsequently, symptomatic [64, 65] and both the WSES and the European Association of Endoscopic Surgery (EAES) advocate appendicectomy in this scenario.

Antibiotic Use

In patients with suspected appendicitis, antibiotics should be started once the pathology is confirmed clinically or radiologically. The topic of surgery versus antibiotics alone has already been discussed earlier. For patients undergoing appendicectomy, broad-spectrum antibiotics given pre-operatively – taking into account local resistance patterns – decrease wound infection and abscess formation [66, 67].

Post-operative use of antibiotics is not recommended for patients who had uncomplicated appendicitis as there is no evidence to support a beneficial effect in this group. Patients with complicated acute appendicitis should receive post-operative broad-spectrum antibiotics [66]. There is no evidence on route and duration of administration, although it appears that 5 days offer no benefit over a 3 day course [68].

Appendix Mass or Abscess

Inflammatory, complicated appendicitis can be in the form of an appendix abscess or phlegmon. This occurs in about 3.8% of patients with appendicitis [69], but does not necessarily follow a delay in diagnosis or treatment [39]. Such pathology can render an appendicectomy very difficult and can lead to resection of the adjoining ileum and/or caecum. Two meta-analyses have shown that the conservative management of complicated appendicitis is associated with a lower complication and re-operation rate and a lower morbidity, when compared to appendicectomy, with a failure of non-surgical treatment in about 7.2% [69, 70]. Antibiotics form the basis of treatment of this group of patients, and drainage of any significant abscess may be required as part of successful conservative management. It is important to exclude malignant disease in patients over 40 as this was detected in 1.2% of cases in one of the meta-analyses [69]. Recurrence rate in the same study was quantified at 7.4%, hence interval appendicectomy would appear to be a reasonable treatment plan to avoid this. However, the morbidity associated with this is as high as 12.4% – with risks such as wound infection, haematoma formation and small bowel obstruction – and this offsets the risk of recurrence. In patients who do get recurrent appendicitis, the WSES recommends interval appendicectomy.

Crohn's Disease

There will be scenarios where an on-table diagnosis of terminal ileal Crohn's disease is made in a patient thought to have acute appendicitis. The decision on whether to resect the pathology or not in these cases is complex and multifactorial – patient factors (nutrition, haemodynamic), disease factors (obstructing pathology, perforation) and surgeon's expertise (colorectal surgeon) are of significant importance.

Appendicitis in Pregnancy

The pregnant patient with right-sided abdominal pain presents a diagnostic dilemma, due to a difficult abdominal examination and potential differential diagnoses such as cholecystitis, as well as the inability to utilise CT as an adjunct in the diagnostic work-up. Surgery is not to be taken lightly because of the risks to the mother and the foetus, but on the other hand complicated appendicitis poses a risk of foetal death or premature labour [71]. Appendicectomy – open or laparoscopic – is the appropriate treatment, however a negative appendicectomy carries a risk to the pregnancy [72].

Appendicitis in Immunocompromised Patients

Immunocompromised patients are susceptible to infection and may not be able to mount an immune response, hence the clinical features in this group of patients are often obtunded. Moreover, biochemical investigations may not be indicative of the ongoing inflammatory process. To compound matters further, pathologies such as neutropenic entercolitis (typhlitis), lymphoma or opportunistic infections may mimic appendicitis. This often leads to delays in diagnosis and hence treatment, with pathology such as established abscess formation creating dilemmas in management as conservative management may fail. CT should be considered early on in these patients, in an attempt to establish the diagnosis and proceed to appendicectomy, if warranted.

Appendiceal Mucinous Neoplasms

A whole spectrum of mucinous neoplasms of the appendix exist, including mucinous cystadenoma, low-grade appendiceal mucinous neoplasm (LAMN) and mucinous cystadenocarcinoma [73]–[75].

Mucinous adenoma is confined to the appendiceal mucosa. It is benign and does not recur. LAMN produces mucin that dissects beyond the appendix, is frequently recurrent, and is associated with low-grade pseudomyxoma peritonei. Mucinous adenocarcinoma is characterised by invasive glands that invade beyond the appendix and are associated with high-grade pseudomyxoma peritonei. Patients with mucinous cystadenocarcinoma have a < 10% 10-year survival.

Mucocoeles are rare, occurring in less than 0.3% of appendicectomy specimens [76, 77]. Only around 50% are symptomatic, with pain, weight loss, nausea and vomiting, abdominal mass or distension being the commonest presenting features [78]. Imaging (US, CT, MRI) may detect mucocoeles or their sequelae.

Management depends on histology, dimensions and the clinical picture. Small mucinous adenomas can be treated with simple appendicectomy. A wide mesoappendix resection is advisable in all cases to allow for lymph node staging, and iatrogenic progression to psuedomyxoma peritonei should be minimised by avoiding perforation of the appendix and/or spillage of contents intra-operatively [79]. Right hemicolectomy is the treatment of choice for invasive adenocarcinoma because of the risk of lymph node involvement [78, 79]. It allows oncologic resection margins, reducing the risk of incomplete clearance. However, it does not confer a survival advantage over simple appendicectomy in patients with peritoneal seeding [80].

Post-Operative Outcomes

Post-operative morbidity specific to appendicectomy arises mainly from surgical site infection (up to 12%), intra-abdominal abscess (up to 8%) and small bowel obstruction (up to 1.9%) [81]–[87]. Management of these cases may range from simple antibiotic therapy, to radiological drainage, to re-laparoscopy or laparotomy.

A diagnosis of appendiceal mucinous tumour is made from histology in between 0.13 and 2.4% of cases, and that of adenocarcinoma in less than 1% of cases [76, 77, 88], with follow-on treatment ranging from none, to resectional surgery with or without hyperthermic intra-peritoneal chemotherapy.

Conclusion

In summary, appendicitis remains a prevalent condition requiring in-hospital management. It has become apparent that the natural history of appendicitis is not the same in all cases, and in fact there may be different pathophysiological processes that dictate the development of uncomplicated or complicated appendicitis. Hence, it is important to classify appendicitis by type, as there may be a role for conservative management in selected cases. Both surgical and interventional techniques have evolved and a tailored management plan should be implemented once staging – or classification – of appendicitis is established.

References

[1] Addiss, DG; Shaffer, N; Fowler, BS; Tauxe, RV. "The epidemiology of appendicitis and appendectomy in the United States.," *Am. J. Epidemiol.*, vol. 132, no. 5, pp. 910–25, Nov. 1990.

[2] Zahid, A. "The vermiform appendix: not a useless organ.," *J. Coll. Physicians Surg. Pak.*, vol. 14, no. 4, pp. 256–8, Apr. 2004.

[3] Bhangu, A; Søreide, K; Di Saverio, S; Assarsson, JH; Drake, FT. "Acute appendicitis: modern understanding of pathogenesis, diagnosis, and management," *Lancet*, vol. 386, no. 10000, pp. 1278–1287, Sep. 2015.

[4] Clanton, J; Subichin, M; Drolshagen, K; Daley, T; Firstenberg, MS. "Fulminant *Clostridium difficile* infection: An association with prior appendectomy?," *World J. Gastrointest. Surg.*, vol. 5, no. 8, p. 233, Aug. 2013.

[5] Frisch, M; Pedersen, BV; Andersson, RE. "Appendicitis, mesenteric lymphadenitis, and subsequent risk of ulcerative colitis: cohort studies in Sweden and Denmark.," *BMJ*, vol. 338, p. b716, Mar. 2009.

[6] Kaplan, GG; Pedersen, BV; Andersson, RE; Sands, BE; Korzenik, J; Frisch, M. "The risk of developing Crohn's disease after an appendectomy: a population-based cohort study in Sweden and Denmark," *Gut*, vol. 56, no. 10, pp. 1387–1392, Oct. 2007.

[7] FITZ, R. "On Perforating Inflammation of the Vermiform Appendix with Special Reference to Its Early Diagnosis and Treatment," *N. Engl. J. Med.*, vol. 213, no. 6, pp. 245–248, Aug. 1935.

[8] Ferris, M; et al., "The Global Incidence of Appendicitis," *Ann. Surg.*, vol. 266, no. 2, pp. 237–241, Aug. 2017.

[9] Anderson, JE; Bickler, SW; Chang, DC; Talamini, MA. "Examining a Common Disease with Unknown Etiology: Trends in Epidemiology and Surgical Management of Appendicitis in California, 1995–2009," *World J. Surg.*, vol. 36, no. 12, pp. 2787–2794, Dec. 2012.

[10] Andersson, RE; Hugander, A; Thulin, AJ. "Diagnostic accuracy and perforation rate in appendicitis: association with age and sex of the patient and with appendicectomy rate.," *Eur. J. Surg.*, vol. 158, no. 1, pp. 37–41, Jan. 1992.

[11] Zingone, F; Sultan, AA; Humes, DJ; West, J. "Risk of Acute Appendicitis in and Around Pregnancy," *Ann. Surg.*, vol. 261, no. 2, pp. 332–337, Feb. 2015.

[12] Carr, NJ. "The pathology of acute appendicitis.," *Ann. Diagn. Pathol.*, vol. 4, no. 1, pp. 46–58, Feb. 2000.

[13] Marudanayagam, R; Williams, GT; Rees, BI. "Review of the pathological results of 2660 appendicectomy specimens," *J. Gastroenterol.*, vol. 41, no. 8, pp. 745–749, Sep. 2006.

[14] Sadr Azodi, O; Andrén-Sandberg, Å; Larsson, H. "Genetic and environmental influences on the risk of acute appendicitis in twins," *Br. J. Surg.*, vol. 96, no. 11, pp. 1336–1340, Nov. 2009.

[15] Ergul, E. "Heredity and Familial Tendency of Acute Appendicitis," *Scand. J. Surg.*, vol. 96, no. 4, pp. 290–292, Dec. 2007.

[16] Lamps, LW. "Infectious Causes of Appendicitis," *Infect. Dis. Clin. North Am.*, vol. 24, no. 4, pp. 995–1018, Dec. 2010.

[17] Gallerani, M; Boari, B; Anania, G; Cavallesco, G; Manfredini, R. "Seasonal variation in onset of acute appendicitis.," *Clin. Ter.*, vol. 157, no. 2, pp. 123–7.

[18] Sesia, S; Mayr, J; Bruder, E; Haecker, FM. "Neurogenic Appendicopathy: Clinical, Macroscopic, and Histopathological Presentation in Pediatric Patients," *Eur. J. Pediatr. Surg.*, vol. 23, no. 03, pp. 238–242, Feb. 2013.

[19] Andersson, REB. "Meta-analysis of the clinical and laboratory diagnosis of appendicitis," *Br. J. Surg.*, vol. 91, no. 1, pp. 28–37, Jan. 2004.

[20] Yu, CW; Juan, LI; Wu, MH; Shen, CJ; Wu, JY; Lee, CC. "Systematic review and meta-analysis of the diagnostic accuracy of procalcitonin, C-reactive protein and white blood cell count for suspected acute appendicitis," *Br. J. Surg.*, vol. 100, no. 3, pp. 322–329, Feb. 2013.

[21] Andersson, M; Rubér, M; Ekerfelt, C; Hallgren, HB; Olaison, G; Andersson, RE. "Can New Inflammatory Markers Improve the Diagnosis of Acute Appendicitis?," *World J. Surg.*, vol. 38, no. 11, pp. 2777–2783, Nov. 2014.

[22] Di Saverio, S; et al., "WSES Jerusalem guidelines for diagnosis and treatment of acute appendicitis," *World J. Emerg. Surg.*, vol. 11, no. 1, p. 34, Dec. 2016.

[23] Ohle, R; O'Reilly, F; O'Brien, KK; Fahey, T; Dimitrov, BD. "The Alvarado score for predicting acute appendicitis: a systematic review.," *BMC Med.*, vol. 9, no. 1, p. 139, Dec. 2011.

[24] Andersson, M; Andersson, RE. "The Appendicitis Inflammatory Response Score: A Tool for the Diagnosis of Acute Appendicitis that

Outperforms the Alvarado Score," *World J. Surg.*, vol. 32, no. 8, pp. 1843–1849, Aug. 2008.

[25] de Castro, SMM; Ünlü, C; Steller, EP; van Wagensveld, BA; Vrouenraets, BC. "Evaluation of the appendicitis inflammatory response score for patients with acute appendicitis.," *World J. Surg.*, vol. 36, no. 7, pp. 1540–5, Jul. 2012.

[26] Kollár, D; McCartan, DP; Bourke, M; Cross, KS; Dowdall, J. "Predicting Acute Appendicitis? A comparison of the Alvarado Score, the Appendicitis Inflammatory Response Score and Clinical Assessment," *World J. Surg.*, vol. 39, no. 1, pp. 104–109, Jan. 2015.

[27] Scott, AJ; Mason, SE; Arunakirinathan, M; Reissis, Y; Kinross, JM; Smith, JJ. "Risk stratification by the Appendicitis Inflammatory Response score to guide decision-making in patients with suspected appendicitis," *Br. J. Surg.*, vol. 102, no. 5, pp. 563–572, Apr. 2015.

[28] Samuel, M. "Pediatric appendicitis score.," *J. Pediatr. Surg.*, vol. 37, no. 6, pp. 877–81, Jun. 2002.

[29] Ebell, MH; Shinholser, J. "What Are the Most Clinically Useful Cutoffs for the Alvarado and Pediatric Appendicitis Scores? A Systematic Review," *Ann. Emerg. Med.*, vol. 64, no. 4, p. 365–372.e2, Oct. 2014.

[30] Florence, M; et al., "Negative Appendectomy and Imaging Accuracy in the Washington State Surgical Care and Outcomes Assessment Program," *Trans. ... Meet. Am. Surg. Assoc.*, vol. 126, no. 4, pp. 198–204, Oct. 2008.

[31] Bachar, I; Perry, ZH; Dukhno, L; Mizrahi, S; Kirshtein, B. "Diagnostic Value of Laparoscopy, Abdominal Computed Tomography, and Ultrasonography in Acute Appendicitis," *J. Laparoendosc. Adv. Surg. Tech.*, vol. 23, no. 12, pp. 982–989, Dec. 2013.

[32] Andersson, RE. "The natural history and traditional management of appendicitis revisited: spontaneous resolution and predominance of prehospital perforations imply that a correct diagnosis is more important than an early diagnosis.," *World J. Surg.*, vol. 31, no. 1, pp. 86–92, Jan. 2007.

[33] Terasawa, T; Blackmore, CC; Bent, S; Kohlwes, RJ. "Systematic review: computed tomography and ultrasonography to detect acute appendicitis in adults and adolescents.," *Ann. Intern. Med.*, vol. 141, no. 7, pp. 537–46, Oct. 2004.

[34] Leeuwenburgh, MMN; et al., "*Accuracy of MRI compared with ultrasound imaging and selective use of CT to discriminate simple from perforated appendicitis on behalf of the OPTIMAP study group*," 2013.

[35] Theilen, LH; et al., "Utility of magnetic resonance imaging for suspected appendicitis in pregnant women," *Am. J. Obstet. Gynecol.*, vol. 212, no. 3, p. 345.e1-345.e6, Mar. 2015.

[36] Atema, JJ; van Rossem, CC; Leeuwenburgh, MM; Stoker, J; Boermeester, MA. "Scoring system to distinguish uncomplicated from complicated acute appendicitis," *Br. J. Surg.*, vol. 102, no. 8, pp. 979–990, Jul. 2015.

[37] Gorter, RR; et al., "Diagnosis and management of acute appendicitis. EAES consensus development conference 2015," *Surg. Endosc.*, vol. 30, no. 11, pp. 4668–4690, Nov. 2016.

[38] Gomes, CA; et al., "Acute appendicitis: proposal of a new comprehensive grading system based on clinical, imaging and laparoscopic findings," *World J. Emerg. Surg.*, vol. 10, no. 1, p. 60, Dec. 2015.

[39] Livingston, EH; Woodward, WA; Sarosi, GA; Haley, RW. "Disconnect Between Incidence of Nonperforated and Perforated Appendicitis," *Ann. Surg.*, vol. 245, no. 6, pp. 886–892, Jun. 2007.

[40] Rubér, M; Andersson, M; Petersson, BF; Olaison, G; Andersson, RE; Ekerfelt, C. "Systemic Th17-like cytokine pattern in gangrenous appendicitis but not in phlegmonous appendicitis," *Surgery*, vol. 147, no. 3, pp. 366–372, Mar. 2010.

[41] Varadhan, KK; Humes, DJ; Neal, KR; Lobo, DN. "Antibiotic Therapy Versus Appendectomy for Acute Appendicitis: A Meta-Analysis," *World J. Surg.*, vol. 34, no. 2, pp. 199–209, Feb. 2010.

[42] Di Saverio, S; et al., "The NOTA Study (Non Operative Treatment for Acute Appendicitis)," *Ann. Surg.*, vol. 260, no. 1, pp. 109–117, Jul. 2014.

[43] Svensson, JF; et al., "Nonoperative Treatment With Antibiotics Versus Surgery for Acute Nonperforated Appendicitis in Children," *Ann. Surg.*, vol. 261, no. 1, pp. 67–71, Jan. 2015.

[44] Salminen, P; et al., "Antibiotic Therapy vs Appendectomy for Treatment of Uncomplicated Acute Appendicitis," *JAMA*, vol. 313, no. 23, p. 2340, Jun. 2015.

[45] Liu, Z; et al., "Laparoscopy or not," *Surg. Laparosc. Endosc. Percutan. Tech.*, vol. 20, no. 6, pp. 362–370, Dec. 2010.

[46] Wei, B; et al., "Laparoscopic versus open appendectomy for acute appendicitis: a metaanalysis," *Surg. Endosc.*, vol. 25, no. 4, pp. 1199–1208, Apr. 2011.

[47] Markar, SR; et al., "Laparoscopic Versus Open Appendectomy for Complicated and Uncomplicated Appendicitis in Children," *J. Gastrointest. Surg.*, vol. 16, no. 10, pp. 1993–2004, Oct. 2012.

[48] Walker, HGM; Al Samaraee, A; Mills, SJ; Kalbassi, MR. "Laparoscopic appendicectomy in pregnancy: A systematic review of the published evidence," *Int. J. Surg.*, vol. 12, no. 11, pp. 1235–1241, Nov. 2014.

[49] Ward, NT; Ramamoorthy, SL; Chang, DC; Parsons, JK. "Laparoscopic appendectomy is safer than open appendectomy in an elderly population.," *JSLS J. Soc. Laparoendosc. Surg.*, vol. 18, no. 3, p. e2014.00322, 2014.

[50] Yeh, CC; Wu, SC; Liao, CC; Su, LT; Hsieh, CH; Li, TC. "Laparoscopic appendectomy for acute appendicitis is more favorable for patients with comorbidities, the elderly, and those with complicated appendicitis: a nationwide population-based study.," *Surg. Endosc.*, vol. 25, no. 9, pp. 2932–42, Sep. 2011.

[51] Jaschinski, T; Mosch, C; Eikermann, M; Neugebauer, EA. "Laparoscopic versus open appendectomy in patients with suspected appendicitis: a systematic review of meta-analyses of randomised controlled trials," *BMC Gastroenterol.*, vol. 15, no. 1, p. 48, Dec. 2015.

[52] Sauerland, S; Jaschinski, T; Neugebauer, EA. "Laparoscopic versus open surgery for suspected appendicitis," *Cochrane Database Syst. Rev.*, no. 10, p. CD001546, Oct. 2010.

[53] Motson, RW; Kelly, MD. "Simplified technique for laparoscopic appendectomy.," *ANZ J. Surg.*, vol. 72, no. 4, pp. 294–5, Apr. 2002.

[54] Street, D; Bodai, BI; Owens, LJ; Moore, DB; Walton, CB; Holcroft, JW. "Simple ligation vs stump inversion in appendectomy.," *Arch. Surg.*, vol. 123, no. 6, pp. 689–90, Jun. 1988.

[55] Lavonius, MI; Liesjärvi, S; Niskanen, RO; Ristkari, SK; Korkala, O; Mokka, RE. "Simple ligation vs stump inversion in appendicectomy.," *Ann. Chir. Gynaecol.*, vol. 85, no. 3, pp. 222–4, 1996.

[56] St Peter, SD; et al., "Irrigation Versus Suction Alone During Laparoscopic Appendectomy for Perforated Appendicitis," *Ann. Surg.*, vol. 256, no. 4, pp. 581–585, Oct. 2012.

[57] Cheng, Y; et al., "Abdominal drainage to prevent intra-peritoneal abscess after open appendectomy for complicated appendicitis," *Cochrane Database Syst. Rev.*, no. 2, p. CD010168, Feb. 2015.

[58] Allemann, P; Probst, H; Demartines, N; Schäfer, M. "Prevention of infectious complications after laparoscopic appendectomy for complicated acute appendicitis--the role of routine abdominal drainage.," *Langenbeck's Arch. Surg.*, vol. 396, no. 1, pp. 63–8, Jan. 2011.

[59] Carter, JT; Kaplan, JA; Nguyen, JN; Lin, MYC; Rogers, SJ; Harris, HW. "A Prospective, Randomized Controlled Trial of Single-Incision Laparoscopic vs Conventional 3-Port Laparoscopic Appendectomy for Treatment of Acute Appendicitis," *J. Am. Coll. Surg.*, vol. 218, no. 5, pp. 950–959, May 2014.

[60] Bingener, J; Ibrahim-zada, I. "Natural orifice transluminal endoscopic surgery for intra-abdominal emergency conditions.," *Br. J. Surg.*, vol. 101, no. 1, pp. e80-9, Jan. 2014.

[61] Chen, J; et al., "Single-incision versus conventional three-port laparoscopic appendectomy: A meta-analysis of randomized controlled trials," *Minim. Invasive Ther. Allied Technol.*, vol. 24, no. 4, pp. 195–203, Jul. 2015.

[62] United Kingdom National Surgical Research Collaborative and A. Bhangu, "Safety of short, in-hospital delays before surgery for acute appendicitis: multicentre cohort study, systematic review, and meta-analysis.," *Ann. Surg.*, vol. 259, no. 5, pp. 894–903, May 2014.

[63] Elniel, M; Grainger, J; Nevins, EJ; Misra, N; Skaife, P. "72h Is the Time Critical Point to Operate in Acute Appendicitis," *J. Gastrointest. Surg.*, vol. 22, no. 2, pp. 310–315, Feb. 2018.

[64] Strong, S; Blencowe, N; Bhangu, A. National Surgical Research Collaborative, "How good are surgeons at identifying appendicitis? Results from a multi-centre cohort study," *Int. J. Surg.*, vol. 15, pp. 107–112, Mar. 2015.

[65] Phillips, AW; Jones, AE; Sargen, K. "Should the Macroscopically Normal Appendix be Removed During Laparoscopy for Acute Right Iliac Fossa Pain When No Other Explanatory Pathology is Found?," *Surg. Laparosc. Endosc. Percutan. Tech.*, vol. 19, no. 5, pp. 392–394, Oct. 2009.

[66] Daskalakis, K; Juhlin, C; Påhlman, L. "The use of pre- or postoperative antibiotics in surgery for appendicitis: A systematic review," *Scand. J. Surg.*, vol. 103, no. 1, pp. 14–20, Mar. 2014.

[67] Andersen, BR; Kallehave, FL; Andersen, HK. "Antibiotics versus placebo for prevention of postoperative infection after appendicectomy.," *Cochrane Database Syst. Rev.*, no. 3, p. CD001439, Jul. 2005.

[68] van Rossem, CC; Schreinemacher, MHF; Treskes, K; van Hogezand, RM; van Geloven, AAW. "Duration of antibiotic treatment after appendicectomy for acute complicated appendicitis," *Br. J. Surg.*, vol. 101, no. 6, pp. 715–719, May 2014.

[69] Andersson, RE; Petzold, MG. "Nonsurgical Treatment of Appendiceal Abscess or Phlegmon," *Ann. Surg.*, vol. 246, no. 5, pp. 741–748, Nov. 2007.

[70] Simillis, C; Symeonides, P; Shorthouse, AJ; Tekkis, PP. "A meta-analysis comparing conservative treatment versus acute appendectomy for complicated appendicitis (abscess or phlegmon)," *Surgery*, vol. 147, no. 6, pp. 818–829, Jun. 2010.

[71] Zhang, Y; Zhao, Y; Qiao, J; Ye, R. "Diagnosis of appendicitis during pregnancy and perinatal outcome in the late pregnancy.," *Chin. Med. J. (Engl).*, vol. 122, no. 5, pp. 521–4, Mar. 2009.

[72] Wilasrusmee, C; Sukrat, B; McEvoy, M; Attia, J; Thakkinstian, A. "Systematic review and meta-analysis of safety of laparoscopic *versus* open appendicectomy for suspected appendicitis in pregnancy," *Br. J. Surg.*, vol. 99, no. 11, pp. 1470–1478, Nov. 2012.

[73] Tirumani, SH; et al., "Mucinous neoplasms of the appendix: a current comprehensive clinicopathologic and imaging review.," *Cancer Imaging*, vol. 13, no. 1, pp. 14–25, Feb. 2013.

[74] Pai, RK; Longacre, TA. "Appendiceal mucinous tumors and pseudomyxoma peritonei: histologic features, diagnostic problems, and proposed classification.," *Adv. Anat. Pathol.*, vol. 12, no. 6, pp. 291–311, Nov. 2005.

[75] Pai, RK; Beck, AH; Norton, JA; Longacre, TA. "Appendiceal Mucinous Neoplasms," *Am. J. Surg. Pathol.*, vol. 33, no. 10, pp. 1425–1439, Oct. 2009.

[76] Chandrasegaram, MD; Rothwell, LA; An, EI; Miller, RJ. "Pathologies of the appendix: a 10-year review of 4670 appendicectomy specimens.," *ANZ J. Surg.*, vol. 82, no. 11, pp. 844–7, Nov. 2012.

[77] In't Hof, KH; van der Wal, HC; Kazemier, G; Lange, JF. "Carcinoid tumour of the appendix: an analysis of 1,485 consecutive emergency appendectomies.," *J. Gastrointest. Surg.*, vol. 12, no. 8, pp. 1436–8, Aug. 2008.

[78] Dixit, A; Robertson, JHP; Mudan, SS; Akle, C. "Appendiceal mucocoeles and pseudomyxoma peritonei.," *World J. Gastroenterol.*, vol. 13, no. 16, pp. 2381–4, Apr. 2007.

[79] Rymer, B; Forsythe, RO; Husada, G. "Mucocoele and mucinous tumours of the appendix: A review of the literature," *Int. J. Surg.*, vol. 18, pp. 132–135, Jun. 2015.

[80] González-Moreno, S; Sugarbaker, PH. “Right hemicolectomy does not confer a survival advantage in patients with mucinous carcinoma of the appendix and peritoneal seeding,” *Br. J. Surg.*, vol. 91, no. 3, pp. 304–311, Mar. 2004.

[81] National Surgical Research Collaborative, “Multicentre observational study of performance variation in provision and outcome of emergency appendicectomy,” *Br. J. Surg.*, vol. 100, no. 9, pp. 1240–1252, Aug. 2013.

[82] Andersson, RE. “Short-term complications and long-term morbidity of laparoscopic and open appendicectomy in a national cohort,” *Br. J. Surg.*, vol. 101, no. 9, pp. 1135–1142, Aug. 2014.

[83] Andersson, REB. “Small bowel obstruction after appendicectomy,” *Br. J. Surg.*, vol. 88, no. 10, pp. 1387–1391, Oct. 2001.

[84] Emil, S; et al., “Determinants of postoperative abscess occurrence and percutaneous drainage in children with perforated appendicitis,” *Pediatr. Surg. Int.*, vol. 30, no. 12, pp. 1265–1271, Dec. 2014.

[85] Fleming, FJ; Kim, MJ; Messing, S; Gunzler, D; Salloum, R; Monson, JR. “Balancing the Risk of Postoperative Surgical Infections,” *Ann. Surg.*, vol. 252, no. 6, pp. 895–900, Dec. 2010.

[86] Guller, U; et al., “Laparoscopic versus open appendectomy: outcomes comparison based on a large administrative database.,” *Ann. Surg.*, vol. 239, no. 1, pp. 43–52, Jan. 2004.

[87] Isaksson, K; Montgomery, A; Moberg, AC; Andersson, R; Tingstedt, B. “Long-term follow-up for adhesive small bowel obstruction after open versus laparoscopic surgery for suspected appendicitis.,” *Ann. Surg.*, vol. 259, no. 6, pp. 1173–7, Jun. 2014.

[88] Charfi, S; Sellami, A; Affes, A; Yaïch, K; Mzali, R; Boudawara, TS. “Histopathological findings in appendectomy specimens: a study of 24,697 cases.,” *Int. J. Colorectal Dis.*, vol. 29, no. 8, pp. 1009–12, Aug. 2014.

Biographical Sketches

Neville Spiteri

Affiliation: Department of Surgery, Aintree University Hospital NHS Foundation Trust

Education: Malta Medical School

Professional Appointments: Clinical Fellow

Honors: MD (Melit) MRCSEd (GenSurg) ChM (GenSurg) FEBS (GenSurg) FRCSEd (GenSurg)

Publications from the Last 3 Years:

Grech N, Ellul E, Spiteri N, Milic M. "Solitary Fibrous Tumour A rare cause of acute abdomen." *Ann Ital Chir.* 2017 Mar 29; 6. pii: S2239253X17026767. PMID: 28904243

Spiteri, Neville. "The impact of stapling technique and surgeon specialism on anastomotic failure after right-sided colorectal resection: An international multi-centre, prospective audit." 2015 European Society of Coloproctology collaborating group. *Colorectal Dis.* 2018 Jun 19. doi: 10.1111/codi.14308. PMID: 29920945

Spiteri, Neville. "The relationship between method of anastomosis and anastomotic failure after right hemicolectomy and ileo-caecal resection: an international snapshot audit." 2015 European Society of Coloproctology collaborating group. *Colorectal Dis.* 2017 Mar 6. doi: 10.1111/codi.13646.

Spiteri, Neville. "Risk factors for unfavourable postoperative outcome in patients with Crohn's disease undergoing right hemicolectomy or ileocaecal resection: An international audit by ESCP and S-ECCO." 2015 European Society of Coloproctology collaborating group. *Colorectal Dis.* 2017 Sep 15. doi: 10.1111/codi.13889. [Epub ahead of print] PMID: 28913968

Spiteri, Neville and Skaife, Paul. "Get FIT for the new year: a review of the role of faecal immunochemical test for haemoglobin in patients with symptoms of colorectal disease." *Journal of Laboratory and Precision Medicine.*2018, 3:52

Paul Skaife

Affiliation: Department of Surgery, Aintree University Hospital NHS Foundation Trust

Education: Leeds Medical School

Professional Appointments: Consultant Colorectal Surgical Oncologist

Honors: MB ChB MD FRCS FRCS (Gen)

Publications from the Last 3 Years:

Altaf, K; Mckernan, G; Skaife, P; Slawik, S. "Splenic metastasis in colorectal cancer." *Tech Coloproctol.*, 2016 Nov, 20(11), 795-796. Epub 2016 Sep 27. No abstract available.

Brown, S; Tiernan, J; Biggs, K; Hind, D; Shephard, N; Bradburn, M; Wailoo, A; Alshreef, A; Swaby, L; Watson, A; Radley, S; Jones, O; Skaife, P; Agarwal, A; Giordano, P; Lamah, M; Cartmell, M; Davies, J; Faiz, O; Nugent, K; Clarke, A; MacDonald, A; Conaghan, P; Ziprin, P; Makhija, R. "The Hubble Trial: haemorrhoidal artery ligation (HAL) versus rubber band ligation (RBL) for symptomatic second- and third-degree haemorrhoids: a multicentre randomised controlled trial and health-economic evaluation." *Health Technol Assess.*, 2016 Nov, 20(88), 1-150.

Elniel, M; Grainger, J; Nevins, EJ; Misra, N; Skaife, P. "72h Is the Time Critical Point to Operate in Acute Appendicitis." *J Gastrointest Surg.*, 2018 Feb, 22(2), 310-315. doi: 10.1007/s11605-017-3614-8. Epub 2017 Oct 30.

Jones CD, Guiot L, Portelli M, Bullen T, Skaife P. "Two Interesting Cases of Meralgia Paraesthetica". *Pain Physician.* 2017 Sep; 20(6):E987-E989. PMID: 28934803

Knowles, CH; Horrocks, EJ; Bremner, SA; Stevens, N; Norton, C; O'Connell, PR; Eldridge, S. "CONFIDeNT study group. Percutaneous tibial nerve stimulation versus sham electrical stimulation for the treatment of faecal incontinence in adults (CONFIDeNT): a double-blind, multicentre, pragmatic, parallel-group, randomised controlled trial." *Lancet*, 2015, Oct 24, 386(10004), 1640-8. doi: 10.1016/S0140-6736(15)60314-2. Epub 2015 Aug 18.

Moug, SJ; Henderson, N; Tiernan, J; Bisset, CN; Ferguson, E; Harji, D. Maxwell-Armstrong C, MacDermid E, Acheson AG, Steele RJC, Fearnhead NS; "The Colorectal Surgeon's personality may influence the rectal anastomotic decision. Edinburgh Delphi Collaborative Group." *Colorectal Dis.* 2018 Jun 14. doi: 10.1111/codi.14293. [Epub ahead of print]

Oldfield, F; Gilbert, T; Skaife, P. "Is modern management of fistula-in-ano acceptable?" *Br J Hosp Med* (Lond)., 2016 Jul, 77(7), 388-93. doi: 10.12968/hmed.2016.77.7.388. Review.

Skaife, Paul. "The impact of stapling technique and surgeon specialism on anastomotic failure after right-sided colorectal resection: An international multi-centre, prospective audit." 2015 European Society of Coloproctology collaborating group. *Colorectal Dis.* 2018 Jun 19. doi: 10.1111/codi.14308. [Epub ahead of print] PMID: 29920945

Skaife, Paul. The relationship between method of anastomosis and anastomotic failure after right hemicolectomy and ileocaecal resection: an international snapshot audit. 2015 European Society of Coloproctology collaborating group. *Colorectal Dis.* 2017 Mar 6. doi: 10.1111/codi.13646. [Epub ahead of print]

Skaife, Paul. Risk factors for unfavourable postoperative outcome in patients with Crohn's disease undergoing right hemicolectomy or ileocaecal resection: An international audit by ESCP and S-ECCO. 2015 European Society of Coloproctology collaborating group. *Colorectal Dis.* 2017 Sep 15. doi: 10.1111/codi.13889. [Epub ahead of print]

In: Appendicitis
Editor: Rose Ballard

ISBN: 978-1-53614-753-7

Chapter 2

AN UPDATE CONCERNING APPENDICITIS: RISK FACTORS AND CLINICAL MANAGEMENT

Kelly Cristine de Lacerda Rodrigues Buzatti[1,*], MD, PhD, Gustavo Monteiro Oliveira[2] and Beatriz Deoti e Silva Rodrigues[2], MD, PhD

[1]Department of Surgery, Faculty of Medicine, Federal University of Minas Gerais, Belo Horizonte, Brazil
[2]Faculty of Medicine, Federal University of Minas Gerais, Belo Horizonte, Brazil

ABSTRACT

Background: Acute appendicitis affects an average of 70,000 American children a year, being the main cause of abdominal surgeries in children. The appendix can be found perforated in up to one third of appendectomies. The diagnosis of appendicitis is based on a history of diffuse abdominal pain, which usually starts in the central region of the abdomen and migrates to the lower right quadrant of the abdomen. It can

* Corresponding Author Email: kellybuzatti@gmail.com, Phone: +55 31 3409-9403 (colorectal surgeon).

vary on its clinical presentation due to the anatomical variation of the vermiform appendix. Appendectomy is still the standard treatment for acute appendicitis but clinical management should be considered in some specific situations.

Aim: The aim of this chapter is to present an updated review chapter of appendicitis regarding its prevalence, risk factors and clinical management.

Method: The chapter was written based on recent articles found on online scientific databases using the keywords: Appendicitis; Prevalence; Risk Factors; Clinical management.

Conclusion: Acute appendicitis is the most common surgical acute disease of the abdominal and has always to be considered in a young patient with abdominal pain. Patients diagnosed with local abscess may require previous clinical treatment before surgery and can be conducted with venous antibiotic therapy and elective appendectomy. Early surgical treatment when appendicitis is complicated with local abscess is associated with higher morbidity compared to initial conservative treatment. Cases of clinical management are exception and all the patients have to be exanimated by a surgeon.

INTRODUCTION

The vermiform appendix is a tubular structure with blind bottom that emerges from the cecum whose function is still unknown. A role in the immune system has already been suggested because of the presence of lymphoid tissue in its structure. However, studies are still needed to confirm this function and to clarify the possible mechanisms involved to immunity. The vermiform appendix has an average diameter of 6 mm and length of 6-8 cm (but can reach 15 cm). The appendix is mainly found in the lower right quadrant of the abdomen. However, its location may vary and it can be found atypically in the pelvis or even on the left side of the abdomen[1-3].

Acute appendicitis is a progressive inflammatory disease of the vermiform appendix that can cause perforation. This condition can be easily identified by inflammatory signs such as vascular congestion, hyperemia and the presence of fibrin in the appendix (Figura 1).

Reginald Fitz first described this abdominal disease in 1886 and the removal of the appendix is still the gold standard treatment since it was described [3].

The luminal obstruction of the appendix may lead to distension and thickening of its wall, which contributes to vascular compression and ischemia. Some agents such as fecaliths, foreign bodies, parasites, lymphoid hyperplasia, and tumors have been described as being responsible for the luminal obstruction of the appendix. Consequently, bacterial invasion and growth may occur which contributes to a more intense inflammatory response, followed by ischemia and necrosis leading to increased risk of perforation. This sequence of events leads to acute appendicitis which may be a life threatening condition if not diagnosed and treated.

Acute appendicitis is frequently associated with a favorable clinical evolution when diagnosed and treated early with antibiotic therapy and surgical intervention. It is the most common cause of abdominal surgery in children and adults admitted to hospital emergencies and it has a peak incidence among patients who are between 10 and 30 years of age. Risk factors for bad outcome are elderly patients with comorbidities, long time of disease evolution and the occurrence of appendicular perforation [4].

Acute appendicitis is an important surgical disease of childhood and affects an average of 70,000 American children per year.

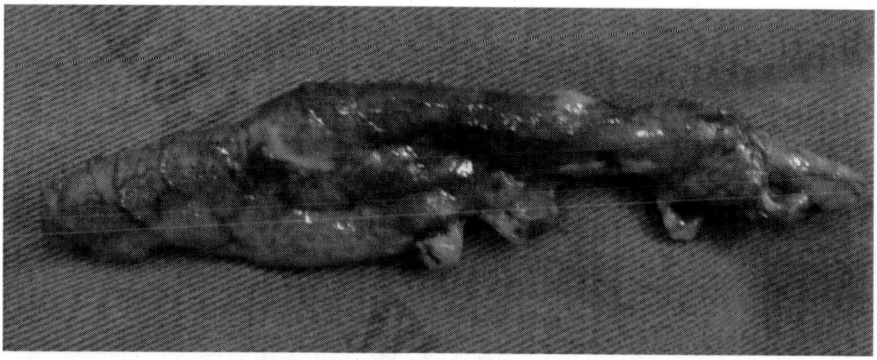

Figure 1. Vermiform appendix with inflammatory signs after appendectomy.

The incidence of appendicitis in the first 4 years of life is 1-6 patients per 10,000 against 19-28 patients per 10,000 in children between 5 and 14 years of age [2, 9].

The diagnosis of acute appendicitis is based on the clinical history of diffuse abdominal pain, which begins in the central region of the abdomen and migrates to the lower right quadrant. It may vary according to the location of the appendix. In general, the abdomen is fragile and sensitive to palpation; abdominal pain may be associated with nausea, vomiting, low fever, high leukocyte count and increased . However, less than 50% of the patients present all these symptoms together. The clinical diagnosis must be confirmed by a surgeon based on the level of clinical suspicion. It can be classified in uncomplicated ou complicated appendicitis (Table 1) [5-8].

Table 1. Acute appendicitis classification [6]

Uncomplicated Appendicitis	**Complicated Appendicitis**
Appendix with increased diameter (usually higher than 10 mm)	Appendix with gangrene and/or perfuration
Inflammatory signs such as vascular congestion, hyperemia and presence of fibrin	Purulent peritoneal liquid
inflammatory process restricted to the right lower quadrant of the abdomen	Intra-abdominal abscess
Potentional non-operative treatment for selected cases	Potentional later appendectomy (interval appendectomy after 8-12 weeks)
Antibiotic prophylaxis	Antibiotic prophylaxis + postoperative antibiotic therapy
Appendectomy as the gold standart treatment	Appendectomy as the gold standart treatment

Despite the well-known clinical history, in atypical cases the diagnosis can be challenging for surgeons. The vermiform appendix may also be found durantion acute appendicitis inside the inguinal hernia sac (Amyand`s hernia), the femoral hernia sac (De Garengeot`s hernia) or in various incisional site abdominal hernias. Another unusual situation occurs in the pregnant woman, in this case physiological and anatomical changes such as the displacement of the appendix to the upper part of the abdomen can make difficult the precise diagnosis [9].

The analysis of blood tests is useful in the diagnosis of appendicitis. The elevated C-reactive protein levels and incresead number of leucocytes seems to increase the accuracy of diagnoses. Blood tests may also be helpful in identifying other causes of acute abdomen such as pancreatitis and cholangitis [6, 10].

Although acute appendicitis is often diagnosed through clinical examination, radiological study is especially useful in cases with atypical clinical course and in the detection of complications associated with this inflammatory process [6]. Ultrasonography of the abdomen (USG) is the first choice method for examination mainly for children and pregnant woman. The normal appendix is found on image examination as a compressible tubular structure with thin wall (less than 2 mm) and diameter up to 10mm. When USG findings are not enough to confirm the diagnosis, the computed tomography (CT) and magnetic resonance imaging are the next step for imaging investigation (Figure 2). Patients who are obese or who are with abdominal distension are not favorable to the USG, then the CT should already be requested as the first method of choice. In addition to the increase in diameter and appendiceal wall, the presence of periapendicular fluid, abscess or fecaliths (Figura 3) are also indicative of an appendicular inflammatory process. In advanced cases with perforation and peritonitis, there may be free fluid in the abdominal cavity.

Clinical mimics such as meckel diverticulitis, cholecystitis, colon diverticulitis, ureterolithiasis and crohn's disease should be considered when the history is not typical or in the presence of chronic symptoms such as diarrhea, weight loss and the presence of blood in the stool.

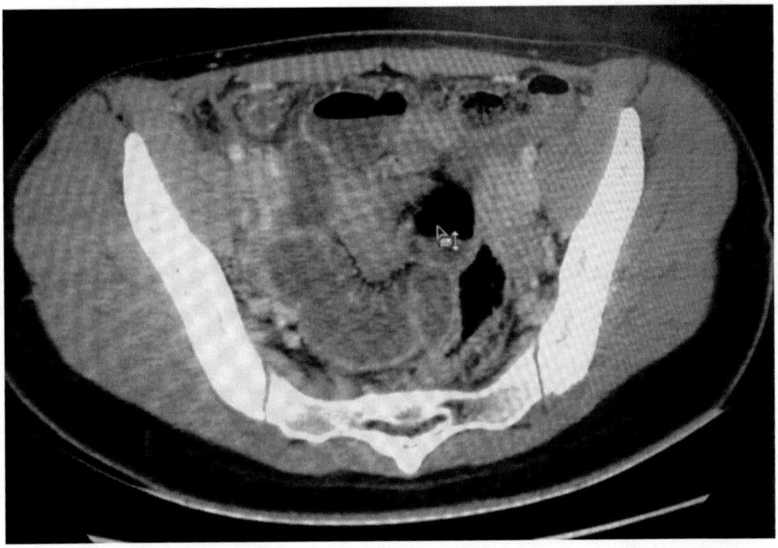

Figure 2. CT imaging scan showing thick and contrast-enhanced appendix wall (arrow).

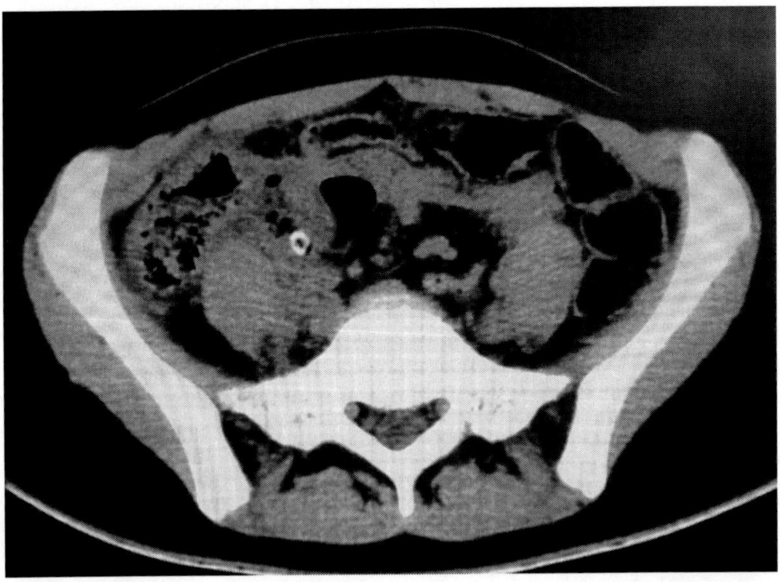

Figure 3. CT imaging scan showing fecalith in the topography of the appendix (arrow).

In women, it may be necessary to make a differential diagnosis with urinary tract infection and inflammatory gynecological diseases. When clinical examination and imaging examination were not sufficient for diagnostic confirmation, laparoscopy should be encouraged in an attempt to avoid late diagnosis and to reduce the incidence of complications and morbidity of this condition [5, 11, 12].

Complicated acute appendicitis occurs after the perforation of the vermiform appendix and it is more common after 72 hours of the onset of the symptoms. In these cases, the clinical course of the disease is quite different from that of uncomplicated acute appendicitis leading to increased risk of postoperative complications and prolonged treatment. Complicated appendicitis has a higher rate of occurrence in the elderly individuals when compared to younger patients, which represents a challenge for surgeons due to the common presence of comorbidities in this age group [9, 13].

Acute appendicitis can also manifest as an appendiceal mass in 2-10% of cases. This finding is usually associated to fever and leukocytosis and it results from the blockade of the appendicular perforated inflammatory process by abdominal viscera and the greater omentum to avoid diffuse peritonitis. In this situation, early surgical treatemnt remains controversial due to the high morbidity and technical difficulty due to adhesions and inflammation process. Another disadvantage of the appendicular mass early approach is the missing of another unexpected disease. Cecal malignancy may be found in 8-15% of the cases of appendiceal mass, another missing diagnosis can be Crohn`s disease, ileal tuberculosis or infection diseases such as actonomycosis [14-16]. The emergency surgery has as advatages the no need for another admission and cost-effective. Most of authors recommend clinical treatment with antibiotics that resolve the inflammatory process in 80% of the cases and later interval appendectomy 8-12 weeks after [13, 16-18].

On the other hand, patients diagnosed with non complicated appendicitis who don`t have diabetes, who are still with short duration of symptoms (< 25 hours), in the absence of appendicolith on imaging examination and with absence of systemic inflammation may even be eligible for non operative treatment. The management of acute appendicitis with antibiotic therapy alone is an alternative treatment to appendectomy for selected patients.

Although some studies have tried to find predictors of success for the conservative treatment, there is a considerable risk of failure with persistence of the inflammatory process, perforation of the appendix or recurrence of the condition. The complications of conservative treatment may even be considered potentially more severe than appendectomy, which justifies the preference for surgical treatment in almost all patients.

Antibiotic prophylaxis is mandatory at the time of the diagnosis in order to prevent surgical site infections and intra-abdominal infectious complications.

Antibiotic treatment should be maintained postoperatively in patients with complicated appendicitis. There has been no literature data to routinely advocate the use of postoperative antibiotic therapy for uncomplicated appendicitis. The choice of the drug should be based on local microbiome and local bacterial resistance patterns. Preoperative management for the surgical procedure should include the administration of antibiotics, fever control, intravascular volumetric replacement, blood glucose adjustment in diabetic patients and immediate initiation of intensive care with cardiac and respiratory monitoring in those patients with severe sepsis. The diet should be suspended until the patient is referred to the surgical block [6, 10, 13, 16].

Discussion

Patients who reach the emergency room with acute appendicitis may have a varied clinical presentation ranging from nonspecific abdominal pain to signs of severity such as peritonitis and sepsis. All patients with abdominal pain or acute abdomen should have as clinical suspicion the inflammation of the appendix until other causes have been identified because of the high prevalence in relation to the other abdominal surgical affections.

Although non-operative treatment of uncomplicated appendicitis has been reported to be able to prevent 60-85% of appendectomies, we advocate appendectomy as the standard gold standard for acute appendicitis untill we have higher qualitative evidence on randomized studies. Furthermore, delaying surgical treatment may lead to progression to complicated appendicitis and increase disease-related morbidity and mortality.

Interval appendectomy is also feasible in cases of complicated appendicitis, when antibiotic therapy and percutaneous drainage of abscesses are performed in the acute phase and the appendectomy is subsequently performed electively. But we still have conflicting results and lack of data to recommend this protocol as routine.

The removal of a normal appendix have been described in up to 15% of appendectomies. The use of available imaging methods should always be encouraged when the clinical setting is not typical. USG is a non-invasive method that is usefull to confirm appendicitis, but it cannot exclude this disease with safety. The USG examination is an operator dependent method and the most common inconclusive radiological finding is not visualizing the appendix. The CT has the disadvantages of using radiation and being a more expensive method, but it is superior to USG with sensitivity and specificity of 76-100% and 83-100%, respectively [6, 10].

Some algorithms such as the Alvarado score that is based on clinical data and biochemical tests were proposed for diagnostic help, but they were not superior to the imaging methods. They may be useful options when radiological exams are not available [6, 10].

CONCLUSION

Acute appendicitis is the most common surgical acute disease of the abdominal and has always to be considered in a young patient with abdominal pain. Patients diagnosed with local abscess may require previous clinical treatment before surgery and can be conducted with venous antibiotic therapy and elective appendectomy. Early surgical treatment when appendicitis is complicated with local abscess is associated with higher morbidity compared to initial conservative treatment. Cases of clinical management are exception and all the patients have to be exanimated by a surgeon.

References

[1] Ceresoli, M., Zucchi, A., Allievi, N., Harbi, A., Pisano, M., Montori, G., et al. Acute Appendicitis: Epidemiology, Treatment and Outcomes- Analysis of 16544 Consecutive Cases. *World journal of gastrointestinal surgery,* 2016; 8(10):693-699.

[2] Prystowsky, J. B., Pugh, C. M., Nagle, A. P. Current Problems in Surgery. Appendicitis. *Current problems in surgery*, 2005; 42(10): 688-742.

[3] Petroianu, A., Villar Barroso, T. V. Pathophysiology of Acute Appendicitis. *JSM Gastroenterol Hepatol.*, 2016; 4(3):1062.

[4] Iamarino, A. P. M., Juliano, Y., Rosa, O. M., Novo, N. F., Favaro, M. L., Ribeiro, M. A. F. J. Risk Factors Associated with Complications of Acute Appendicitis. *Revista do Colegio Brasileiro de Cirurgioes*, 2017; 44(6):560-566.

[5] Wray, C. J., Kao, L. S., Millas, S. G., Tsao, K., Ko, T. C. Acute Appendicitis: Controversies in Diagnosis and Management. *Current problems in surgery*, 2013; 50(2):54-86.

[6] Gorter, R. R., Eker, H. H., Gorter-Stam, M. A., Abis, G. S., Acharya, A., Ankersmit, M., et al. Diagnosis and Management of Acute Appendicitis. Eaes Consensus Development Conference 2015. *Surgical endoscopy*, 2016; 30(11):4668-4690.

[7] Alvarado, A. How to Improve the Clinical Diagnosis of Acute Appendicitis in Resource Limited Settings. *World journal of emergency surgery : WJES,* 2016; 11:16.

[8] Choksuwattanasakul, M. Incidental Appendectomy During Mini Incision Post-Partum Sterilization (Chokchai Technique): A Prospective Cross-Sectional Study. *The journal of obstetrics and gynaecology research,* 2017.

[9] Demir, M. K., Savas, Y., Furuncuoglu, Y., Cevher, T., Demiral, S., Tabandeh, B., et al. Imaging Findings of the Unusual Presentations, Associations and Clinical Mimics of Acute Appendicitis. *The Eurasian journal of medicine,* 2017; 49(3):198-203.

[10] Shogilev, D. J., Duus, N., Odom, S. R., Shapiro, N. I. Diagnosing Appendicitis: Evidence-Based Review of the Diagnostic Approach in 2014. *The western journal of emergency medicine*, 2014; 15(7):859-871.

[11] Debnath, J., Sharma, V., Ravikumar, R., Kumar, R., Chatterjee, S., Sampath, S., et al. Clinical Mimics of Acute Appendicitis: Is There Any Role of Imaging? *Medical journal, Armed Forces India*, 2016; 72(3):285-292.

[12] Mostbeck, G., Adam, E. J., Nielsen, M. B., Claudon, M., Clevert, D., Nicolau, C., et al. How to Diagnose Acute Appendicitis: Ultrasound First. *Insights into imaging*, 2016; 7(2):255-263.

[13] Cohen-Arazi, O., Dabour, K., Bala, M., Haran, A., Almogy, G. Management, Treatment and Outcomes of Acute Appendicitis in an Elderly Population: A Single-Center Experience. *European journal of trauma and emergency surgery : official publication of the European Trauma Society*, 2016.

[14] Castro, L. L., Cabral, M. M. D. Á., Andrade, R. F. M., Buzatti, K. C. d. L. R., Silva, R. G. d. Actinomycosis Mimicking Colonic Neoplasia. *Journal of Coloproctology (Rio de Janeiro),* 2012; 32:312-315.

[15] Joshi, D. S., Fleming, A. E., Spottswood, S. E. It's Not Appendicitis? Consideration of a Benign Mimicker. *Hospital pediatrics*, 2015; 5(2):101 - 105.

[16] Demetrashvili, Z., Kenchadze, G., Pipia, I., Ekaladze, E., Kamkamidze, G. Management of Appendiceal Mass and Abscess. An 11-Year Experience. *International surgery*, 2015; 100(6):1021-1025.

[17] Campbell, M. R., Johnston, S. L. 3rd., Marshburn, T., Kane, J., Lugg, D. Nonoperative Treatment of Suspected Appendicitis in Remote Medical Care Environments: Implications for Future Spaceflight Medical Care. *Journal of the American College of Surgeons*, 2004; 198(5):822-830.

[18] Andersson, R. E., Petzold, M. G. Nonsurgical Treatment of Appendiceal Abscess or Phlegmon: A Systematic Review and Meta-Analysis. *Annals of surgery,* 2007; 246(5):741-748.

In: Appendicitis
Editor: Rose Ballard

ISBN: 978-1-53614-753-7

Chapter 3

RECURRENT/STUMP APPENDICITIS

Al Giwa[1,*], Nathan Louras[1] and Demis Lipe[2]
[1]Department of Emergency Medicine
Icahn School of Medicine at Mount Sinai, New York, NY, US
[2]Martin Army Community Hospital, Fort Benning, GA, US

ABSTRACT

The residual remnant or "stump" of the appendix after an initial appendectomy may become inflamed causing what is commonly referred to as stump appendicitis. The incidence of stump appendicitis is estimated to be 1 in 50,000 cases, making the diagnosis exceedingly rare. This uncommon disease coupled with a prior history of appendectomy can lead to a delay in diagnosis. While no single cause has been identified, there is evidence to suggest that the length of the residual stump after resection has an influence on recurrent infection. The difficulty in the diagnosis of the disease lies in its ambiguous presentation in the setting of a presumed completely resected appendix. Unfortunately, giving the often nonspecific vital signs and inconclusive laboratory results as the initial available data, a physician will need to maintain a high clinical suspicion in order to make the correct diagnosis. The use of computed tomography (CT) scans has reduced the need for more invasive diagnostic techniques and aids in the physician's ability to expeditiously diagnose stump appendicitis.

* Corresponding Author Email: Al.Giwa@MountSinai.org.

Ultrasonography has also been demonstrated to aid in the diagnosis of stump appendicitis, particularly where CT scans are not as readily available. Treatment with antibiotics may be attempted as an alternative to surgery; however, the vast majority of cases require definitive surgical excision of the remnant appendix. Stump appendicitis is a problematic disease with an underestimated prevalence. Delays in diagnosis can lead to significant patient morbidity and more complex surgical procedures. Keeping this disease in the differential is important in reducing complications associated with delayed diagnosis.

INTRODUCTION/EPIDEMIOLOGY

Recurrent, or as it is more commonly referred to in the surgical literature, stump appendicitis is a rare complication post appendectomy, which could have detrimental consequences if not diagnosed in a timely manner. Stump appendicitis is an inflammation or obstruction of the residual appendiceal tissue after an appendectomy and has been associated with the length of the residual stump (Liang, Lo, and Marks 2006). The first description of stump appendicitis was provided by T. F. Rose in 1945 (Rose 1945). Since that time, the incidence of stump appendicitis has been estimated to be 1 in 50,000 cases (Mangi and Berger 2000). A more recent study found a total of 5 stump appendicitis cases out of 3130 patients who underwent appendectomy making the incidence closer to 0.16% (Dikicier et al. 2018). However, these numbers are likely to be an underestimate as many cases of stump appendicitis go unreported throughout the world and the condition is poorly defined.

A review of the more recent studies looking at stump appendicitis revealed a total of 61 case reports in the English literature (Geraci et al. 2016, Kanona et al. 2012, Subramanian and Liang 2012, Maurice et al. 2016). The age range for recurrence has been shown to be from 8 to 72 years of age, with a mean age of 35 +/- 2 years (Geraci et al. 2016). The disease process favors men over women with a male to female ratio of 1:1.7 (Leff et al. 2012, Geraci et al. 2016, Maurice et al. 2016). Lastly, the time interval between initial operation and re-operation was between 4 days and 50 years, with the average time to recurrence being reported to be 108 months, making this potentially a part of the post-appendectomy differential for the remainder of a person's life (Geraci et al. 2016, Giwa and Reyes 2018, Mangi and Berger 2000, Liang, Lo, and Marks 2006). As reported by Giwa and Reyes, it is important to remember that having one recurrence of stump appendicitis does not rule out the possibility of another recurrence, as their patient presented to the Emergency Department after 2 prior appendectomies with yet another case of stump appendicitis.

Many of medicine's most respected authors and some of the standard textbooks in Emergency Medicine and General Surgery have failed to adequately discuss the possibility of a recurrence of appendicitis in patients post appendectomy. There is not a single mention of recurrent or stump appendicitis in Tintinalli, Cameron, Greenfield, Sabiston, Rosai and Ackerman, or O' Leary; all major texts in Emergency Medicine and General Surgery. The only textbooks that provide any significant information on stump appendicitis are Schwartz's Principles of Surgery (Liang et al. 2014) followed by Rosen's Emergency Medicine, which provides 2 sentences on the subject (Cole and Huang 2018). This chapter aims to collate the information available on the differential of right lower quadrant pain irrespective of prior appendectomy and highlight the current literature surrounding stump appendicitis. We will discuss presentation, diagnostic evaluation, and treatment of this rare disease process.

PATHOPHYSIOLOGY

Embryologically, the appendix is a continuation of the cecum and can measure up to 20 centimeters (cm) long, however on average the appendix measures approximately 10cm. Its base is located posterior-medially to the cecum and about 2.5 to 3cm below the ileocecal valve. While the etiology of stump appendicitis is unclear, obstruction of a long appendiceal stump with a fecalith or fecal stasis has been attributed to stump appendicitis. The obstruction will cause increased mucous production, which in turn leads to increased pressure which leads to bacterial overgrowth. The increasing intraluminal pressure leads to distention of the stump causing visceral pain, followed by peritoneal irritation from ongoing edema. (Levine, 2017) Non-obstructive inflammation of the appendiceal stump can also occur. This inflammation can cause venous congestion and in return, increases intraluminal pressure (Garden and Parks 2018).

While it has been proposed that stump appendicitis is a problem that is unique to and increased with the use of laparoscopic procedures, this theory has not been substantiated by any independent body or literature review (Subramanian and Liang 2012). Some surgeons suggest a higher incidence of stump appendicitis after open appendectomy; however, this may be due to the number of open procedures performed worldwide versus laparoscopically since the first reported case of stump appendicitis in 1945 (Giwa and Reyes 2018, Johnston, Myers, and Williams 2015). Some authors have also argued that the laparoscopic approach increases the risk of stump appendicitis due to the smaller field of vision and absence of tactile feedback (Ismail et al. 2009)), again there is little data to support this.

Some of the first reported cases of stump appendicitis occurred in the 1940's long before the routine use of laparoscopy (Rose 1945) (Baumgardner 1949). Research by Liang et al. did not support a statistically significant increase in incidence of recurrent appendicitis after laparoscopic vs. open appendectomy (Giwa and Reyes 2018) (Liang, Lo, and Marks 2006). In fact, they found at the time of their literature review, that of the 36 total cases of stump appendicitis studied, 34% were laparoscopic whereas 66% were open laparotomies (Giwa and Reyes 2018) (Liang, Lo, and Marks 2006). Much of the current data has shown the correlation between the length of the remaining appendix and recurrence of infection. A long appendiceal stump of greater than 0.5cm has been the most commonly cited etiologic factor in stump appendicitis (Gasmi et al. 2009) (Subramanian and Liang 2012) (Liang, Lo, and Marks 2006), however, complicated appendicitis at initial presentation has also been cited as a contributing factor due to the increased difficulty in dissecting the appendix (Subramanian and Liang 2012). The long stump can lead to inflammation or obstruction with a fecalith, which can in turn cause stump appendicitis. Fistulas, masses, and abscesses have all been documented complications associated with stump appendicitis (Tang et al. 2011) (Rose 1945). The inability of the surgeon to clearly distinguish the appendix from its surrounding structures may lead to incomplete resection. Misleading cecum base identification due to edema, abscesses or abnormal anatomical position of the appendix as well as multiple adhesions around the site are also contributing factors (Belli et al. 2011).

A delay in the diagnosis coupled with a low index of suspicion have been factors attributed to the high perforation rate of stump appendicitis. Continued luminal pressure can eventually lead to venous obstruction, thrombosis and arterial compromise. The pathophysiologic changes will in turn lead to gangrene and perforation (Al Mansour and Watch 2011).

Clinical Presentation

The signs and symptoms of stump appendicitis are very similar to acute appendicitis (Truty et al. 2008) (Maurice et al. 2016). The most common presenting symptom is abdominal pain, which makes the differential very broad. The location of the appendix, and therefore the stump, determines the presenting signs and symptoms. Not unlike cases of acute (primary) appendicitis, the appendiceal stump may be located retrocecal or retroileal, in the pelvis or be low lying. A gravid uterus may also displace the appendix superiorly, thereby mimicking gall bladder disease (Manfredi and Ranniger 2013). Patients tend to have a myriad of other symptoms including nausea, vomiting, diarrhea, or hematochezia. However, the overwhelming majority will present with acute or chronic abdominal pain (Subramanian and Liang 2012). Certain conditions may obscure the diagnosis of stump appendicitis, such as extremes of age, mental retardation, immunosuppression and steroid use (Gupta et al. 2000).

Children may present with atypical signs and symptoms, as well as the typical right lower quadrant pain and related gastrointestinal symptoms. Initial presentations in pediatrics have been reported to range from mild erythema at the incision site to fistulas developed on the abdominal wall from the tip of the stump. The perforation rate in children, has been reported to be approximately 60% and often this is the manner in which children will present to a medical provider, i.e., with peritonitis and severe signs of toxicity (Tang et al. 2011) (Schreiner et al. 2013).

Pregnant patients may also present atypically due to the anatomic and physiologic changes of pregnancy. While maternal death is rare from appendicitis itself, perforation from the stump may cause peritonitis and increase fetal mortality. Stump appendicitis in pregnant patients may present as preterm labor and/or delivery, chorioamnionitis or tubal abscess (Belli et al. 2011).

DIFFERENTIAL DIAGNOSIS

The differential diagnosis is similar to that of acute appendicitis and includes infectious colitis, neutropenic typhlitis, Crohn's disease, epiploic appendagitis, Meckel's diverticulum, as well as urinary tract diseases, such as complicated urinary tract infections, urolithiasis and gynecologic causes of lower abdominal pain. It is important to bear in mind that children, pregnant women and the elderly may have an atypical presentation and simply present with peritonitis.

Table 1. Differential Diagnosis of Right Lower Quadrant Pain After Appendectomy (Watkins, Kothari, and Landercasper 2004)

Cecal Diverticulitis	Meckel's diverticulitis
Regional enteritis	Abdominal wall hematoma
Ureteral stone	Seminal vesiculitis
Psoas abscess	Pelvic inflammatory disease
Prostatitis	Acute Testicular Disease
Incarcerated Hernia	Mesenteric Ischemia
Ovarian torsion	Mittelschmerz
Regional enteritis	Ectopic Pregnancy
Pyelonephritis	Rectus Muscle Strain
Herpes Zoster	Sickle Cell Crisis
Cholecystitis	Perinephric Abscess
Crohn's disease	Omental Torsion
Mesenteric Adenitis	Symptomatic Aortic or Iliac Aneurysm

Diverticulum of the cecum is a rare typically benign condition that manifests itself after hemorrhagic or inflammatory complications (Karatepe et al. 2008). It is worth noting that cecal diverticulitis might be clinically indistinguishable from acute appendicitis. The diagnosis is often made intraoperatively as it is difficult to make preoperatively, unless imaging is done. CT scan is the most sensitive imaging study to date, but ultrasound has also been used with a reported sensitivity of 91.3% and specificity of 99.8% and an overall accuracy greater than 99% in the diagnosis of cecal diverticulitis (Karatepe et al. 2008). Table 1 shows a broad differential for right lower quadrant pain after undergoing appendectomy.

COMPLICATIONS

Appendectomy, whether from primary appendicitis or recurrent appendicitis has been known to be associated with a number of complications. The complication rate increases significantly when the appendix is perforated or gangrenous. Some of the complications can have severe morbidity and increase the mortality rate. Multiple recurrences of stump appendicitis as reported in the literature can lead to increased risk of surgical complications (Giwa and Reyes 2018).

Enterocutaneous fistula is a rare, but known complication post-appendectomy. The condition is associated with increased morbidity and mortality. Fistula formation can be due to many etiological factors, such as leakage from the stump, inflammatory bowel disease, tumors or obstruction. Any one of these factors can lead to fistula formation at any point, postoperatively. Depending on the patient's condition at the time of presentation, an enterocutaneous fistula might be treated surgically or with conservative management. Fistulography should be considered as a diagnostic adjunct in this special scenario, if CT scan does not confirm or rule out the diagnosis (Agostinho, Bains, and Sardelic 2017) (Tang et al. 2011).

Superficial wound infection post-operatively is a common appendectomy complication as well as a stump appendicitis presentation.

Wound erythema has been cited along with abdominal pain as a sign of stump appendicitis (Tang et al. 2011) (Belli et al. 2011).

The presence of an appendiceal abscess is another common complication. Many patients will have a fever and leukocytosis in the setting of right iliac fossa pain. This clinical presentation makes the decision to pursue further investigation with the use of imaging techniques more likely, thus leading to an earlier diagnosis. Appendiceal abscesses can lead to more interventions including drain placement, intraoperative washouts or intravenous antibiotics requiring hospital admission. All of which, may prolong a patient's length of stay in the hospital (Awe, Soliman, and Gourdie 2013) (Van Paesschen et al. 2017).

Perforation of the appendix, whether primary or recurrent, while not a direct complication of appendectomy is often how children and the elderly will present. Perforation of the stump will cause high morbidity and mortality in this population. It is believed that the high rate of perforation in children younger than five years of age is due to the presence of a short, incompletely formed omentum. While in the elderly, a thinner, atrophic and more vulnerable appendix is often the cause of perforation (Durgun et al. 2003). The rate of perforation approaches 68% in stump appendicitis (Ekici et al. 2016).

DIAGNOSIS

Making the diagnosis of stump appendicitis can be challenging given the vague presentation of the abdominal symptoms. In addition to the history and physical exam, physicians can use a combination of laboratory exams and imaging techniques to aid in their evaluation of the patient. However, no single laboratory test is sufficient in making the diagnosis of stump appendicitis. It is reasonable to engage a general surgeon early in the presentation if the patient presents with an acute surgical abdomen or when the suspicion of stump appendicitis is high. Unfortunately, the greatest hurdle to making the diagnosis of stump appendicitis is overcoming the anchoring bias of the previous appendectomy, and not accepting the possibility of a recurrence (Giwa and Reyes 2018) (Awe, Soliman, and Gourdie 2013) (Roberts et al. 2011). Many case reports on stump appendicitis demonstrate normal vital signs without fever or tachycardia on presentation (Ismail et al. 2009) (Karaisli et al. 2017) (Shah et al. 2017) (Harris 1989). Roberts et al. demonstrated a mean white blood cell count on presentation in a reported 40 cases to be 13,700 cells/mm^3 (range, 8 to 27,000) (Roberts et al. 2011). In a select few cases, C-reactive protein was elevated, however this is not routinely measured in the work-up of abdominal pain and is non-specific at best (Ismail et al. 2009) (Karaisli et al. 2017). Urinalysis was also consistently normal in the cases reviewed (Ismail et al. 2009) (Karaisli et al. 2017) (Shah et al. 2017). However, as stated above, the presence of an intraabdominal abscess may present with both a fever and elevated white blood cell count.

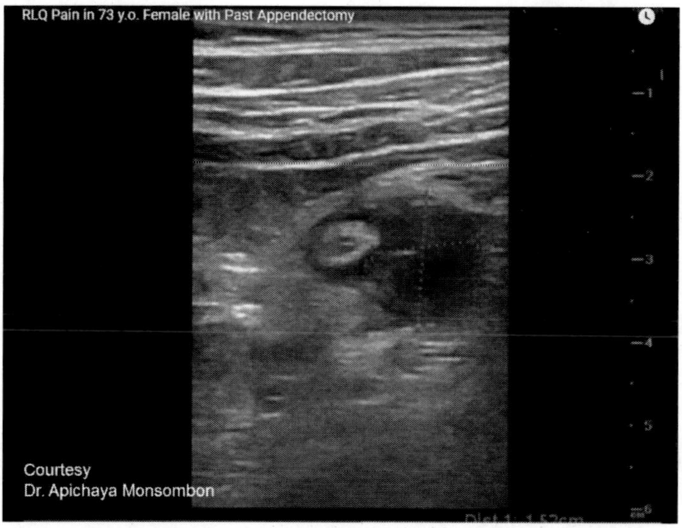

Figure 1. Ultrasound image shows a short axis view of the appendix with a periappendiceal fluid collection measuring approximately 1.5 cm in diameter (73 year-old female who underwent appendectomy 27 years earlier who presented with acute abdominal pain).

There is little radiologic literature when it comes to stump appendicitis due to its rarity (Johnston, Myers, and Williams 2015). However, radiographic imaging is important in establishing the diagnosis of stump appendicitis, as the clinical exam and laboratory work-up can be non-specific. In many resource poor areas of the world, ultrasound is the imaging modality of choice, as it is inexpensive and usually more available than computed tomography. Operators of the ultrasound may find a hypoechoic mass with free fluid in the right iliac fossa. (See Figures 1 and 2. Figure 3 is the confirmatory CT of the same case). Ismail et al., argue that stump appendicitis may be diagnosed with ultrasound alone. The use of graded compression (Puylaert's technique) and identification of an aperistaltic segment of bowel in the right lower quadrant may aid the operator in the diagnosis of stump appendicitis (Puylaert 1986) (Ciftci, Abdurrahman, and Tatar 2015).

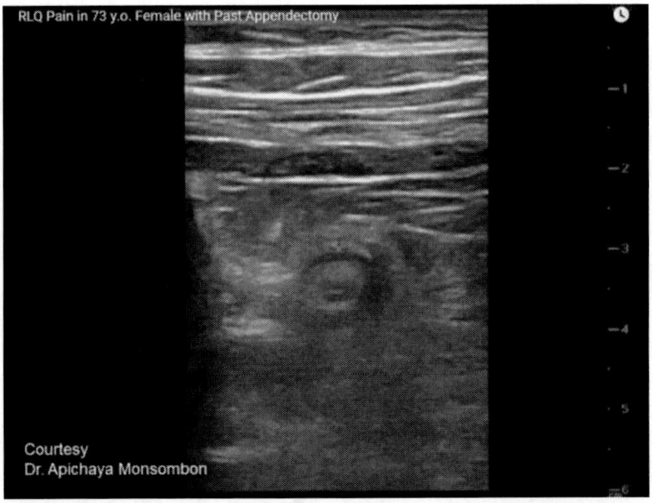

Figure 2. Ultrasound image with a short axis view of the appendix with periappendiceal fluid (73 year-old female who underwent appendectomy 27 years earlier who presented with acute abdominal pain).

More invasive techniques have also been used, though not as commonly given the risk of morbidity. Diagnostic laparoscopy has been described as a definitive diagnostic approach. This modality is both diagnostic and therapeutic, as the surgeon has the option to intervene in the appropriate scenario (Shah et al. 2017) (Watkins, Kothari, and Landercasper 2004). In resource poor areas where patients may be required to be transferred to a different facility for imaging, laparoscopy may be the safest diagnostic mode. The use of colonoscopy has also been described in the work-up of stump appendicitis (Ciftci, Abdurrahman, and Tatar 2015) (Geraci et al. 2016). This is typically used in older patients with vague or atypical abdominal complaints suggestive of possible inflammatory bowel disease. In such cases, identification of a fecalith at the appendicular orifice with surrounding cecal inflammatory changes establishes the diagnosis.

The most frequently used imaging technique described in the literature has been computed tomography (CT) scan (Watkins, Kothari, and Landercasper 2004). CT scanning also provides for a more comprehensive evaluation of the abdomen while being less invasive. Many of the findings are similar to acute appendicitis such as pericecal fat stranding, pelvic abscess, or inflammatory changes of the proximal cecum (Watkins, Kothari, and Landercasper 2004). (See Figures 3 to 5). Findings specifically suggestive of stump appendicitis are the presence of an appendiceal stump with a diameter greater than 6 mm (Johnston, Myers, and Williams 2015). In addition, the presence of either an appendicolith or inflammatory changes surrounding a blind-ended tubular structure at the base of the cecum is pathognomonic for stump appendicitis (Watkins, Kothari, and Landercasper 2004) (Maurice et al. 2016). While the position of the stump and cecum can vary, the relationship between the appendix and the cecum is constant, at approximately 3cm below the ileocecal valve. This fact must be kept in mind when attempting to identify the appendiceal stump on CT scan. It is important to not misinterpret the terminal ileum as the appendiceal stump (Martinez Chamorro et al. 2013).

It is imperative to keep in mind that there are radiologic mimics of stump appendicitis as reported by Johnston et al. Tubo-ovarian abscess, malignancy, para-tubal endometriosis and ileitis may all radiologically mimic stump appendicitis. It is important to take a thorough history and perform a detailed physical exam, including a genital exam if warranted. Crohn's disease, diverticulitis and epiploic appendagitis may also share similar radiologic features. In stump appendicitis, imaging should demonstrate a stump arising from the cecum and terminating at the level of the appendectomy sutures (Johnston, Myers, and Williams 2015). Histopathology of the tissue itself will confirm the diagnosis.

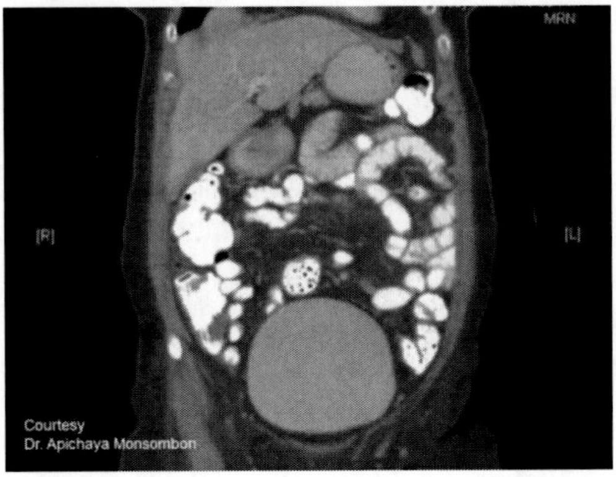

Figure 3. Confirmatory computed tomography (CT) scan of above referenced ultrasounds showing coronal view with the arrow identifying a hollow viscous structure adjacent to the cecum consistent with the residual (stump) appendix (73 year-old female who underwent appendectomy 27 years earlier who presented with acute abdominal pain).

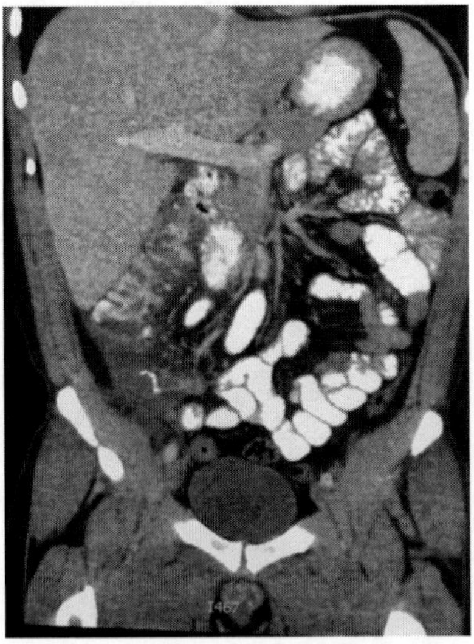

Source: Case courtesy of Demis Lipe, MS, MD, FACEP.

Figure 4. Coronal view of computed tomography scan demonstrates inflammatory region in the right lower quadrant with phlegmonous changes.

The utilization of appropriate diagnostic modalities for stump appendicitis is important to reduce complications in this disease. The consequences of a delayed diagnosis can have significant negative effects for the patient.

Treatment

Definitive treatment for stump appendicitis is the removal of the infected segment of appendix that remains. This is typically done using either an open or a laparoscopic technique. The question of how to manage the appendiceal stump during surgery has been debated for many years. Mayo advocated the use of simple ligation in the primary appendectomy and this has been advocated in the management of the recurrent appendix (Ismail et al. 2009) (Sinha 1977), while others believed that inverting the stump into the cecum after ligation was the safest way to prevent postoperative complication. The reason being that the inverted stump would reduce exposure of the surrounding structures to the contaminated intraluminal surface of the newly ligated stump, as well as minimize the likelihood of intra-abdominal bleeding from the ligated appendiceal artery (Sinha 1977). To date, there has been no data to support the superiority of one technique over the other, including the use of Endoloops, stump inversion, angled endoscopes or EndoGIA stapling devices (Leff et al. 2012) (Mangi and Berger 2000) (Watkins, Kothari, and Landercasper 2004). Other studies have found an association between the length of stump and stump appendicitis. A stump length of 3-5 millimeters has been reported as the standard to minimize postoperative complications. Stumps longer than 5 millimeters may serve as a receptacle for fecoliths (Ismail et al. 2009) (Mangi and Berger 2000) (Ciftci, Abdurrahman, and Tatar 2015).

During the surgical procedure, the surgeon should always obtain the critical view of the appendix, which involves visualizing the attachment of the appendix at the base of the cecum, as well as view the termination of the taenia coli at the base of the appendix (Subramanian and Liang 2012) (Maurice et al. 2016). Dissection and ligation of the recurrent branch of the appendiceal artery marks the true base of the appendix, ensuring adequate removal of the appendiceal tissue (Roche-Nagle et al. 2005). The variable position of the appendix in relation to the cecum and terminal ileum, in addition to localized inflammation, can make obtaining the critical view difficult. Failure to view the base of the appendix due to inflammation, perforation, or phlegmon can lead to misidentification of the appendix-cecum junction. This in turn may cause incomplete or partial resection of the appendix (Maurice et al. 2016) (Ismail et al. 2009).

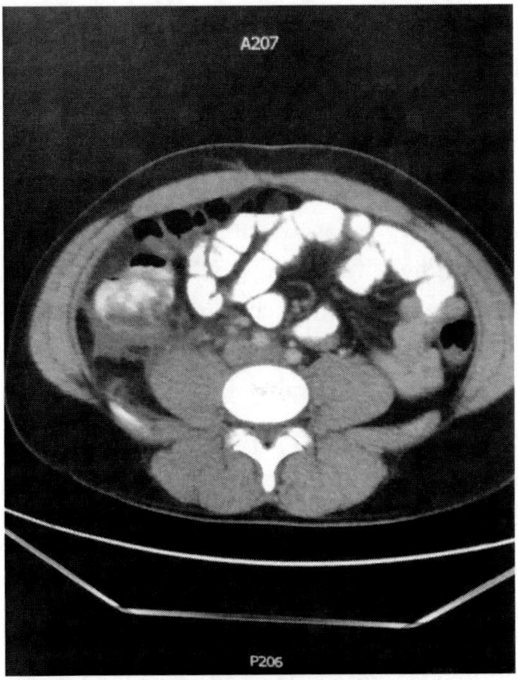

Source: Case courtesy of Demis Lipe, MS, MD, FACEP.

Figure 5. Axial view of computed tomography scan showing phlegmonous process surrounding the prior appendectomy site.

In some instances, this incomplete resection may result in a more morbid procedure (Harris 1989) (Lin et al. 2009) (Mangi and Berger 2000). A review of 60 cases of stump appendicitis, by Leff et al., showed that 13.3% required ileo-cecectomy, in other words, the removal of just the remnant appendiceal stump was not sufficient. Additionally, 10 of the 60 cases required either cecal resection or ileo-cecectomy (Leff et al. 2012). It cannot be overstated that all surgeries ultimately have an effect on a patient's quality of life. While shared decision making with the patient ensures that there is a documented discussion of the benefits and the risks, when returning to the operating room the sum total of all surgeries bear some form of morbidity for the patient.

The effect on each patient is demonstrated in the overall length of stay (LOS) after undergoing surgery. The average LOS after undergoing surgery for stump appendicitis was 10.3 days, compared to a median of 3 days LOS for primary appendectomies (Leff et al. 2012).

In some instances, treatment with antibiotics alone has been used due to the clinical status of the patient. In such cases, the antibiotics of choice were a combination of ciprofloxacin and metronidazole (Giwa and Reyes 2018) (Lipe 2018). In one report, clindamycin was substituted for ciprofloxacin due to allergies. However, in other cases, patients are admitted for observation during the trial of medical management with intravenous antibiotics. In many cases however, conservative management was unsuccessful and required the patients to return to the operating room for definitive surgical treatment (Leff et al. 2012) (Jacombs, Webb, and Leibman 2008). Due to the limited amount of reported cases, there is not enough data to accurately draw conclusions on the effectiveness of medical management on the treatment of stump appendicitis.

Conclusion

Stump appendicitis is a rare and often overlooked disease in patients with prior history of appendectomy. The signs and symptoms are similar to those of acute appendicitis, and share a broad differential in the work-up of their abdominal pain. Concern clearly lies with a delay in diagnosis. This tends to occur when the disease process is not considered, which may lead to complications such as perforation and sepsis. In the absence of a clear clinical picture, CT scan of the abdomen and pelvis provides the most comprehensive image in the least invasive manner. Completion appendectomy should be performed, either with the open or laparoscopic technique. The critical view should be obtained prior to removal of the appendiceal stump and a stump length no longer than 5 millimeters should remain. Medical management with antibiotics is increasingly becoming more common in the these cases and is a reasonable approach if in-patient observation or hospitalization is available, and close follow-up can be assured in a reliable patient.

REFERENCES

Agostinho, N., Bains, H. K. & Sardelic, F. (2017). "Enterocutaneous Fistula Secondary to Stump Appendicitis." *Case Rep Surg*, 6135251. doi: 10.1155/2017/6135251.

Al-Dabbagh, A. K., Thomas, N. B. & Haboubi, N. (2009). "Stump appendicitis. A diagnostic dilemma." *Tech Coloproctol*, *13* (1), 73-4. doi: 10.1007/s10151-008-0419-5.

Al Mansour, Mazen. & Libby, Watch. (2011). "Granulomatous Stump Appendicitis Mimicking Crohn's Disease." *The American Surgeon*, *77* (8), E172-174.

Awe, J. A., Soliman, A. M. & Gourdie, R. W. (2013). "Stump appendicitis: an uncompleted surgery, a rare but important entity with potential problems." *Case Rep Surg*, 972596. doi: 10.1155/2013/972596.

Baumgardner, L. O. (1949). "Rupture of appendiceal stump 3 months after uneventful appendectomy with repair and recovery." *Ohio State Med J*, *45* (5), 476.

Belli, Sedat, Cem, Yalcinkaya, Ali, Ezer, Filiz, Bolat., Tamer, Colakoglu. & Erhan, S, Msek. (2011). "Stump appendicitis and chorioamnionitis due to incomplete appendectomy: A case report." *The Turkish Journal of Gastroenterology*, *22* (5), 540-543. doi: 10.4318/tjg.2011.0265.

Ciftci, F., Abdurrahman, I. & Tatar, Z. (2015). "Stump Appendicitis: A Clinical Enigma." *Chirurgia (Bucur)*, *110* (6), 562-4.

Cole, Michael A. & Robert, D Huang. (2018). "Acute Appendicitis." In *Rosen's Emergency Medicine: Concepts and Clinical Practice*, edited by Ron M. Walls, Robert S. Hockberger and Marianne Gausche-Hill. Philadelphia, PA: Elsevier, Inc.

Dikicier, E., Altintoprak, F., Ozdemir, K., Gundogdu, K., Uzunoglu, M. Y., Cakmak, G., Onuray, F. & Capoglu, R. (2018). "Stump appendicitis: a retrospective review of 3130 consecutive appendectomy cases." *World J Emerg Surg*, *13*, 22. doi: 10.1186/s13017-018-0182-5.

Durgun, A. V., Baca, B., Ersoy, Y. & Kapan, M. (2003). "Stump appendicitis and generalized peritonitis due to incomplete appendectomy." *Tech Coloproctol*, *7* (2), 102-4. doi: 10.1007/s10151-003-0018-4.

Ekici, M. F., Bayhan, Z., Zeren, S., Ucar, B. I., Korkmaz, M. & Deger, A. N. (2016). "A serious conundrum for surgeons: Stump appendicitis." *North Clin Istanb*, *3* (3), 237-239. doi: 10.14744/nci.2016.21043.

Garden, O. James. & Rowan, W. Parks. (2018). *Principles and Practice of Surgery*, 7th ed. Vol. 12. Edinburgh: Elsevier.

Gasmi, M., Fitouri, F., Sahli, S., Jemai, R. & Hamzaoui, M. (2009). "A stump appendicitis in a child: a case report." *Ital J Pediatr*, *35* (1), 35. doi: 10.1186/1824-7288-35-35.

Geraci, G., Di Carlo, G., Cudia, B. & Modica, G. (2016). "Stump appendicitis. A case report." *Int J Surg Case Rep*, *20*, 21-3. doi: 10.1016/j.ijscr.2015.12.049.

Giwa, A. & Reyes, M. (2018). "Three times a charm... a case of repeat appendicitis status post two prior appendectomies." *Am J Emerg Med*, *36* (3), 528 e1-528 e2. doi: 10.1016/j.ajem.2017.12.024.

Gupta, Rajesh, Joel, Gernshiemer, Jonathan, Golden., Nagarjun, Narra. & Timothy, Haydock. (2000). "Abdominal Pain Secondary to Stump Appendicitis in a Child." *The Journal of Emergency Medicine*, *18* (4), 431-433.

Harris, C. R. (1989). "Appendiceal stump abscess ten years after appendectomy." *Am J Emerg Med*, *7* (4), 411-2.

Ismail, I., Iusco, D., Jannaci, M., Navarra, G. G., Grassi, A., Bonomi, S., Parpanesi, R., Giombi, A. & Virzi, S. (2009). "Prompt recognition of stump appendicitis is important to avoid serious complications: a case report." *Cases J*, *2*, 7415. doi: 10.4076/1757-1626-2-7415.

Jacombs, A., Webb, G. & Leibman, S. (2008). "Right iliac fossa pain 10 years after appendicectomy and the diagnosis of stump appendicitis." *ANZ J Surg*, *78* (8), 711-2. doi: 10.1111/j.1445-2197.2008.04624.x.

Johnston, J., Myers, D. T. & Williams, T. R. (2015). "Stump appendicitis: surgical background, CT appearance, and imaging mimics." *Emerg Radiol*, *22* (1), 13-8. doi: 10.1007/s10140-014-1253-x.

Kanona, H., Al Samaraee, A., Nice, C. & Bhattacharya, V. (2012). "Stump appendicitis: a review." *Int J Surg*, *10* (9), 425-8. doi: 10.1016/j.ijsu.2012.07.007.

Karaisli, S., Bag, H., Kar, H., Celik, S. C. & Genc, H. (2017). "Stump Appendicitis: Result of an Incomplete Surgery." *Turk J Gastroenterol*, *28* (3), 223-224. doi: 10.5152/tjg.2017.17082.

Karatepe, O., Gulcicek, O. B., Adas, G., Battal, M., Ozdenkaya, Y., Kurtulus, I., Altiok, M. & Karahan, S. (2008). "Cecal diverticulitis mimicking acute Appendicitis: a report of 4 cases." *World J Emerg Surg*, *3*, 16. doi: 10.1186/1749-7922-3-16.

Leff, D. R., Sait, M. R., Hanief, M., Salakianathan, S., Darzi, A. W. & Vashisht, R. (2012). "Inflammation of the residual appendix stump: a systematic review." *Colorectal Dis*, *14* (3), 282-93. doi: 10.1111/ j.1463-1318.2010.02487.x.

Levine, E. A. & Mowery, N. (2017). "Diseases of appendix." Mulholland MW, Lillemoe KD, Doherty GM, et al., eds. *Greenfield's Surgery: Scientific Principles and Practice*. 6th ed. Philadelphia: Wolters Kluwer; Chap 71.

Liang, M. K., H. G. Lo, and J. L. Marks. 2006. "Stump appendicitis: a comprehensive review of literature." *Am Surg*, *72* (2), 162-6.

Liang, Mike K., Roland, E. Andersson., Bernard, M. Jaffe. & David, H. Berger. (2014). "The Appendix." In *Schwartz's Principles of Surgery, 10e*, edited by F. Charles Brunicardi, Dana K. Andersen, Timothy R. Billiar, David L. Dunn, John G. Hunter, Jeffrey B. Matthews and Raphael E. Pollock. New York, NY: McGraw-Hill Education.

Lin, C. T., Kuo, S. M., Wu, C. C. & Jao, S. W. (2009). "Unusual right upper quadrant Stump Appendicitis." *Z Gastroenterol*, *47* (9), 819-21. doi: 10.1055/s-0028-1109422.

Lipe, Demis. (2018). "Gone but Not Forgotten: Acute Appendicitis Postappendectomy." *Emergency Medicine*, *50*(4), 98-100. doi: 10.12788/emed.2018.0089.

Manfredi, Rita A. & Claudia, Ranniger. (2013). "Appendicitis." In *Emergency Medicine*, edited by James Adams, 325-330. Philadelphia, Pa: Elsevier/Saunders.

Mangi, A. A. & Berger, D. L. (2000). "Stump appendicitis." *Am Surg*, *66* (8), 739-41.

Martinez Chamorro, E., Merina Castilla, A., Munoz Fraile, B., Koren Fernandez, L. & Borruel Nacenta, S. (2013). "Stump appendicitis: preoperative imaging findings in four cases." *Abdom Imaging*, *38* (6), 1214-9. doi: 10.1007/s00261-013-0008-6.

Maurice, A. P., Ibrahim, H., Franz, R. & Iswariah, H. (2016). "Stump appendicitis 5 years after laparoscopic appendicectomy." *BMJ Case Rep*. doi: 10.1136/bcr-2016-217022.

Puylaert, J. B. (1986). "Acute appendicitis: US evaluation using graded compression." *Radiology*, *158* (2), 355-60. doi: 10.1148/radiology. 158.2.2934762.

Richmond, B. (2011). "The appendix." Townsend CM Jr, Beauchamp RD, Evers BM, Mattox KL, eds. *Sabiston Textbook of Surgery: The Biological Basis of Modern Surgical Practice*. 20th ed. Philadelphia: Elsevier; 2017. 1296-311.

Roberts, K. E., L. F. Starker, A. J. Duffy, R. L. Bell, and J. Bokhari. "Stump appendicitis: a surgeon's dilemma." *JSLS*, *15* (3), 373-8. doi: 10.4293/108680811X13125733356954.

Roche-Nagle, G., Gallagher, C., Kilgallen, C. & Caldwell, M. (2005). "Stump appendicitis: a rare but important entity." *Surgeon*, *3* (1), 53-4.

Rose, T. F. (1945). "Recurrent appendiceal abscess." *Medical Journal of Australia*, *32*, 659-662.

Schreiner, Cynthia., Jr. Charles, W. Hartin., Sani, Z. Yamout., Doruk, E. Ozgediz. & Philip, L. Glick. (2013). "A Warning: Don't Be Stumped by Stump Appendicitis." *Pediatric Emergency Care*, *29* (1), 76-77.

Shah, T., Gupta, R. K., Karkee, R. J. & Agarwal, C. S. (2017). "Recurrent pain abdomen following appendectomy: Stump Appendicitis, a surgeon's dilemma." *Clin Case Rep, 5* (3), 215-217. doi: 10.1002/ccr3.781.

Sinha, A. P. (1977). "Appendicectomy: an assessment of the advisability of stump invagination." *Br J Surg, 64* (7), 499-500.

Subramanian, A. & Liang, M. K. (2012). "A 60-year literature review of stump appendicitis: the need for a critical view." *Am J Surg, 203*, (4), 503-7. doi: 10.1016/j.amjsurg.2011.04.009.

Tang, X. B., Qu, R. B., Bai, Y. Z. & Wang, W. L. (2011). "Stump appendicitis in children." *J Pediatr Surg, 46* (1), 233-6. doi: 10.1016/ j.jpedsurg.2010.09.049.

Truty, M. J., Stulak, J. M., Utter, P. A., Solberg, J. J. & Degnim, A. C. (2008). "Appendicitis after appendectomy." *Arch Surg, 143* (4), 413-5. doi: 10.1001/archsurg.143.4.413.

Van Paesschen, C., Haenen, F., Bestman, R. & Van Cleemput, M. (2017). "Stump appendicitis 10 years after appendectomy, a rare, but serious complication of appendectomy, a case report." *Acta Chir Belg, 117* (1), 49-51. doi: 10.1080/00015458.2016.1199353.

Watkins, B. P., Kothari, S. N. & Landercasper, J. (2004). "Stump appendicitis: case report and review." *Surg Laparosc Endosc Percutan Tech, 14* (3), 167-71.

Biographical Sketches

Demis N. Lipe, MD, FAAEM

Affiliation: US Army – Martin Army Community Hospital – Emergency Department, Fort Benning, GA
Piedmont at Columbus Regional – Emergency Department, Columbus, GA

Education: Dr. Lipe received her medical degree from New Jersey Medical School in Newark, NJ in 2011. Prior to obtaining her medical degree, she received a Master of Science in Chemical Biology from Stevens Institute of Technology and her Bachelor of Arts from Rutgers University.

Research and Professional Experience: Dr. Lipe is currently an officer and emergency physician in the United States Army. She trained in Fort Hood, Texas and was then assigned to the Emergency Department Fort Benning in Georgia. Here she served as the director of Trauma and MASCAL Services, as well as assistant professor for Military/Emergency Medicine in association with the Uniformed Services University of the Health Sciences (USUHS), F. Edward Hebert School of Medicine. She has also spent her time doing telemedicine, which is a professional interest.

Dr. Lipe's academic interest include, out-of-hospital cardiac arrest, telemedicine, oncologic emergencies and physician wellbeing. She is a fellow of American Academy of Emergency Medicine and member of the wellness committee. She is also a peer reviewer for high impact journals such as Annals of Emergency Medicine.

Professional Appointments: Assistant Professor for Military/Emergency Medicine in association with the Uniformed Services University of the Health Sciences (USUHS), F. Edward Hebert School of Medicine.

Publications from the Last 3 Years:

Hurst, NB; Lipe, DN; Karpen, S; Patanwala, A; Boesen, KJ; Shirazi, FM. "Centuroides sculpturatus envenomation in three adult patients requiring treatment with antivenom." *Clin Toxicol*, 2018, 56(4), 294-296. PMID: 28871821.

Lipe DN. "Gone but not forgotten. Acute Appendicitis Post Appendectomy." *Emergency Medicine*, 2018, 50(4), 98-100.

Lipe, DN and Affleck, S. "Atypical Presentation of Hand, Foot, and Mouth in an Adult." *Clin Pract Cases Emerg Med*, 2018, 2(2), 179-180. DOI: 10.5811/cpcem.2018.3.37686.

Lipe, DN. "An Emergency Physician's Perspective on Army Medicine." *Mil Med*, 2018, 183(5-6), 113-114. PMID: 29548005.

Lipe, DN. "Infant with a Diffuse Rash and a Fever." *Ann Emerg Med*, 2018, 71(2), 263,270. PMID: 29447868.

Lipe, DN. "Young woman with a blue, painful and swollen arm." *Ann Emerg Med*, 2017, 70(6), 922,936. PMID: 29157693.

Lipe, DN and Cuthbert, D. "Approach to the multi-trauma patient with sternoclavicular dislocation." *Emergency Medicine*, 2017, 49(8), 364-368. DOI:10.12788/emed.2017.0047.

Lipe, DN and Cuthbert, D. "Rare Case of Unilateral Phlegmasia Cerulea Dolens with Bilateral Deep Vein Thrombosis at a Community Military Hospital Emergency Department." *Mil Med*, 2017, 182(5), e1823-e1825. DOI: 10.7205/MILMED-D-16-00346. PMID: 29087934.

Lipe, DN and Borden, N. "Rare Radiological Pattern of Diffuse Esophageal Spasm." *West J Emerg Med*, 2015, 16(3), 426–427. DOI:10.5811/westjem.2015.3.25826. PMID: 25987921.

Lipe, DN, Lindstrom, R; Tauferner, D; Mitchell, C; Moffett, P. "An Evaluation of Karl Storz CMAC Tip Device versus Traditional Means of Airway Suction In A Cadaveric Model." *West J Emerg Med*, 2014, 15(4), 548-553. DOI: 10.5811/westjem.2014.3.21646. PMID: 25035766.

Al O. Giwa, LLB, MD, MBA, FAAEM, FACEP

Affiliation: Icahn School of Medicine at Mount Sinai

Education: University of Ilorin (LLB), Columbia University College of Physicians and Surgeons (MD), George Washington University (MBA), Clarkson University (MS Bioethics)

Research and Professional Experience: Dr. Giwa has been practicing Emergency Medicine for over 20 years. In addition to his academic interests he has served in various administrative roles at various institutions ranging from Assistant and Associate Medical Director to department Chairman. He has also served as Program Director of the Emergency Medicine residency program and the Director of Clinical Operations at Saint Michael's Medical Center in Newark, NJ. He has consulted in and out of healthcare as the Primary and Senior Consultant of Giwa and Associates Consulting providing risk management, ethics, operational and management consulting services. He is an officer in the US Army where he was until recently the Medical Director for the Combat Medic Instructors program, and is currently part of a Forward Resuscitative Surgical Team.

His specific medical interests are Law and Ethics in Healthcare, Combat Medicine, Resuscitation/Critical Care in the Emergency Department and Difficult Airway Management. He is a member of the Mount Sinai Ethics Committee, a fellow of the American Academy of Emergency Medicine and American College of Emergency Physicians, an editor of several peer reviewed journals in critical care, trauma, and emergency medicine, and board certified by the American Board of Emergency Medicine.

Professional Appointments: Assistant Professor Department of Emergency Medicine Icahn School of Medicine at Mount Sinai; Assistant Professor Department of Emergency Medicine at Seton Hall School of Medicine.

Publications from the Last 3 Years:

Giwa, A. "A Case of Primary Adrenal Failure in the Emergency Department". *American Journal of Emergency Medicine*. (PubMed ID: 29066187).

Giwa, A. Healthcare Ethics and the Law- A Review Article on Why Law Pervades Medicine. *Journal of Community Medicine*- Editorial Issue. 2018; 2: 1007. Open Access: http://meddocsonline.org/journal-of-community-medicine/Healthcare-ethics-and-the-law-Why-law-pervades-medicine.pdf.

Giwa, A. The Right to Die: An Analysis on the Current Laws Banning Physician Aid in Dying Statutes in New York State. *Journal of Medicine and Law*

Giwa, A; Murphy, C. Update article on Influenza: Challenges in Diagnosis and Management in the Emergency Department. *Emergency Medicine Practice*.

Giwa, A; Nguyen, M. "Late onset postpartum preeclampsia: Is it time to reconsider if it's really too late? - A case of preeclampsia 3 months after delivery". *American Journal of Emergency Medicine*. (PubMed ID: 28712641).

Giwa, A; Oey, E. "The Return of an Old Nemesis: Survival after Severe Tricyclic Antidepressant Toxicity". *Toxicology Reports*. (PubMed ID: 29854605).

Giwa, A; Reyes, M. "Three Times A Charm- Recurrent Appendicitis Status Post Two Prior Appendectomies". *American Journal of Emergency Medicine*, (PubMed ID: 29269161).

Nathan J Louras

Affiliation: Mount Sinai Medical Center

Education: Emergency Medicine Resident at Mount Sinai Medical Center, University of Vermont Medical School

Research and Professional Experience: Postdoctoral Research Fellow at the Center for Transplantation Sciences at Massachusetts General Hospital

Professional Appointments: Emergency Medicine Resident

Publications from the Last 3 Years:

[1] Louras, N; Fortune, J; Osler, T; Hyman, N. "Nontrauma surgeons can safely take call at an academic, rural level I trauma center." *American Journal of Surgery,* 2016, Jan, 211(1), 129-132. Cited in PubMed; PMID: 26318915.

[2] Patel, MS; Louras, NJ; Vagefi, PA. "Liver xenotransplantation." *Current Opinion of Organ Transplantation,* 2017, Aug, 10(1097), 459. Cited in PubMed; PMID: 28817400.

[3] Shah, JA; Patel, MS; Elias, N; Navarro-Alvarez, N; Rosales, I; Wilkinson, RA; Colvin, RB; Louras, NJ; Hertl, M; Fishman, JA; Cosimi, AB; Markmann, JF; Sachs, DH; Vagefi, PA. "Prolonged Survival Following Pig-to-Primate Liver Xenotransplantation Utilizing Exogenous Coagulation Factors and Co-Stimulation Blockade." *American Journal of Transplant,* 2017, Jun, 17(8), 2178-2185. Cited in PubMed; PMID: 28489305.

[4] Sahara, H; Sekijima, M; Ariyoshi, Y; Kawai, A; Miura, K; Waki, S; Louras, N; Tomita, Y; Nakano, K; Matsunari, H; Date, H; Nagashima, H; Shimizu, A; Yamada, K. "Effects of Carbon Monoxide on Early Dysfunction and Microangiopathy Following GalT-KO Porcine Pulmonary Xenotransplantation in Cynomolgus Monkeys." *Xenotransplantation*, 2017, Oct 25, Cited in PubMed; PMID: 29067747.

[5] Wang, Z; Louras, NJ; Lellouch, AG; Pratts, SG; Zhang, H; Wang, H; Huang. CA; Madsen, JC; Sachs, DH; Wang, Z. "Dosing optimization of CCR4 immunotoxin for improved depletion of CCR4+ Treg in Non-Human Primates." *Molecular Oncology,* 2018, Jun 5, Cited in Pubmed; PMID: 29873181.

BIBLIOGRAPHY

Acute appendicitis in pregnancy

LCCN	2010037324
Type of material	Book
Personal name	Augustin, Goran.
Main title	Acute appendicitis in pregnancy / Goran Augustin, Mate Majerovic.
Published/Created	Hauppauge, N.Y.: Nova Biomedical Books, c2011.
Description	39 p.: ill.; 22 cm.
ISBN	9781611225815 (softcover)
LC classification	RG580.A6 A94 2011
Related names	Majerovic, Mate.
Contents	Incidence -- History taking and clinical examination -- Examination -- Differential diagnosis -- Diagnostic tests -- Negative appendectomy -- Management -- Prognosis.
Subjects	Pregnancy--Complications. Appendicitis. Pregnancy Complications. Abdomen, Acute. Appendicitis.

Notes Includes bibliographical references (p. [31]-39) and index.
Series Pregnancy and infants: medical, psychological and social issues

American Academy of Pediatrics textbook of adolescent health care
LCCN 2010915359
Type of material Book
Main title American Academy of Pediatrics textbook of adolescent health care / editor in chief, Martin M. Fisher; coeditors, Elizabeth M. Alderman, Richard E. Kreipe, Walter D. Rosenfield.
Published/Created [Elk Grove Village, Ill.]: American Academy of Pediatrics, c2011.
Description xxxvi, 2010 p.: ill. (some col.); 28 cm.
Links Publisher description http://www.loc.gov/catdir/enhancements/fy1205/2010915359-d.html
ISBN 9781581102697
1581102690
LC classification RJ550 .A46 2011
Other title Textbook of adolescent health care
Textbook of adolescent care
Related names Fisher, Martin.
Alderman, Elizabeth M.
Kreipe, Richard E.
Rosenfeld, Walter D.
American Academy of Pediatrics.
Contents History of adolescent medicine and health care -- Epidemiology of mortalities and morbidities in adolescents -- International adolescent health -- Normal pubertal physical growth and development -- Adolescent brain and cognitive changes -- Adolescent psychosocial development

and behavior -- Adolescent sexual development -- Medical history -- Physical examination and laboratory screening -- The approach to symptoms in the adolescent patient -- Legal and ethical issues in adolescent health care -- Adherence issues -- Screening in adolescent health care -- Immunizations -- Anticipatory guidance -- Adolescent nutrition and physical activity -- Complementary and alternative medicine -- Pain in adolescents: pathophysiology and management -- Palliative care and psychological aspects of death and dying in adolescence -- Pharmacologic considerations -- Health policy and financing for adolescent and young adult health services -- The adolescent-friendly practice -- Documentation, coding, and billing -- The adolescent in-patient unit -- School-based health care -- College health -- Health care of incarcerated adolescents -- Health care of adolescents in military settings -- Adolescents in foster care -- Immigrant adolescents -- Transition of adolescents with special health care needs to adulthood -- Solid organ transplantation -- Communication between parents and adolescents -- Parenting the adolescent -- Divorce, separation, and blended families -- Adoption and adolescence -- Adolescents with lesbian or gay parents -- Family systems approaches to adolescent health and illness -- Peers -- Socioeconomic status -- The media -- Computers, technology, and the internet -- Cultural considerations in adolescent health care -- Religion and spirituality -- Cults and adolescents -- Environmental health -- Adolescents at work -- Disasters -- Adolescent sexual behaviors -- Issues affecting gay, lesbian, and bisexual youth -- Medical treatment of the transgender adolescent -- Contraception -- Sexually transmitted infections -- Adolescent pregnancy -- Adolescent parenthood -- Abortion in adolescents -- Sexual dysfunction -- Physiology of menstruation -- Perineal and vaginal abnormalities -- Cervical findings and the papanicolaou smear -- The uterus and adnexa -- Amenorrhea -- Menstrual disorders: dysmenorrhea and premenstrual syndrome -- Abnormoral uterine bleeding -- Hyper-androgenism -- Breast disorders in the female -- Pubertal gynecomastia -- Disorders of the male genitalia -- Growth disorders -- Disorders of puberty -- Pituitary disorders -- Thyroid disorders in adolescents -- Diabetes mellitus -- Adrenocortical disorders -- Bone health and disorders -- Anorexia nervosa -- Bulimia nervosa -- The female athlete triad -- Obesity -- Chest pain in adolescents -- Hyperlipidemia and atherosclerosis -- Congenital heart disease -- Carditis in the adolescent -- Valvular heart diseases -- Cardiac dysrhythmias -- Sudden cardiac death -- Shock in the adolescent patient -- Upper respiratory tract infections -- Lower respiratory infections -- Asthma -- Vocal cord dysfunction in adolescents -- Cystic fibrosis -- Sleep disorders -- Pneumothorax -- Pulmonary embolism -- The approach to abdominal pain -- Functional GI disorders -- Disorders of the esophagus -- Peptic ulcers and other disorders of the stomach and duodenum -- Disorders of the liver and pancreas -- Diseases of the gallbladder -

- Appendicitis -- Diarrhea in the adolescent -- Inflammatory bowel disease -- Celiac disease -- Disorders of the red blood cells Sickle cell disease -- Hemostasis and thrombosis -- White blood cell disorders in adolescents -- Lymphadenopathy and splenomegaly -- Malignant solid tumors -- Brian tumors in adolescents -- Hematopoietic stem cell (bone marrow) transplantation -- Cancer survival issues -- Proteinuria and hematuria -- Urinary tract infections -- Nephritis and nephrosis -- Hypertension: significance, diagnosis, and management -- Voiding disorders -- Systemic lupus erythematosus -- Juvenile idiopathic arthritis -- Vasculitis and associated illnesses -- Fibromyalgia syndrome in adolescents -- Chronic fatigue syndrome -- Central nervous system infections -- Headaches -- Seizures in adolescents -- Motor unit disorders -- Movement disorders and ataxia -- Demyelinating diseases -- CNS trauma -- Intracranial vascular malformations -- Myelomeningocele -- Altered states of consciousness -- Fever of unknown origin -- Common viral infections in adolescents -- Infectious mononucleosis and mononucleosis-like syndromes -- HIV and AIDS in adolescents -- Bacterial infections -- Tick-borne diseases -- Mycobacterial -- Parasitic infections -- Prevention of travel-related infections -- Acne -- Dermatitis and papulosquamous diseases -- Alopecia -- Miscellaneous dermatologic disorders in adolescence -- Genetic disorders -- Genetic predisposition to common disorders -- Special issues of genetic testing in adolescent patients --

Environmental allergies -- Food allergies -- Immunodeficiencies -- Eye disorders -- ENT disorders -- Medical and psychosocial considerations for the deaf adolescent -- Adolescent oral health -- Disorders of the upper extremities -- Disorders of the lower extremities -- Bone and joint infections -- Bone tumors -- Disorders of the spine -- Chest wall abnormalities -- Preparticipation evaluation -- Rehabilitation and strength training -- Exertional heat-related illnesses -- Sport psychology -- Physical abuse -- Sexual abuse and assault -- Prostitution and sex trafficking -- Adolescents in gangs -- Overview: substance abuse -- Tobacco -- Alcohol -- Marijuana -- Stimulants -- Opiates -- Hallucinogens, club drugs, inhalants, and other substances of abuse -- Abuse of prescription drugs -- Overdose of prescription drugs -- Office management and laboratory testing -- Treatment options -- Somatoform disorders in adolescents -- Mood disorders in adolescents -- Disorders of anxiety in adolescents -- Disorders of behavior -- Personality disorders in adolescents -- Psychotic disorders in adolescents -- Psychiatric emergencies in adolescents -- Adolescent psychopharmacology -- Mental health treatment modalities for adolescents -- Neuropsychologic testing of adolescents -- Academic overachievement and underachievement -- Psychoeducational assessment of adolescents -- Gifted adolescents -- ADHD in adolescents.

Subjects Adolescent medicine.
Adolescent psychology.
Teenagers--Health and hygiene.

	Adolescent Medicine.
	Adolescent Psychology.
	Adolescent.
Notes	At head of title: American Academy of Pediatrics.
	Includes bibliographical references and index.

Appendicitis: risk factors, management strategies and clinical implications

LCCN	2014944805
Type of material	Book
Main title	Appendicitis: risk factors, management strategies and clinical implications / Angela S. Marmo, editor.
Published/Produced	New York: Nova Biomedical, [2014]
Description	xvii, 296 pages: illustrations; 26 cm.
ISBN	9781633215269 (hbk.)
	1633215261 (hbk.)
LC classification	MLCM 2018/47747 (R)
Related names	Marmo, Angela S., editor.
Subjects	Appendicitis.
Notes	Includes bibliographical references and index.
Series	Emergency and intensive care medicine

Appendicitis: symptoms, diagnosis, and treatments

LCCN	2010031736
Type of material	Book
Main title	Appendicitis: symptoms, diagnosis, and treatments / William L. Ryan, editor.
Published/Created	New York: Nova Science Publisher's, c2010.
Description	xi, 151 p: ill.; 26 cm.
ISBN	9781617617379 (hardcover)
LC classification	RD542 .A67 2010
Related names	Ryan, William L., 1964-

Contents	Appendicitis: symptoms, diagnosis, and treatments / Andy Petroianu -- Acute appendicitis in pregnancy / Goran Augustin, Mate Majerovic -- Appendicitis: symptoms, diagnosis, and treatments / Laura Armañanzas, Jaime Ruiz-Tovar, Rafael Calpena -- Antibiotic therapy alone in the management of acute appendicitis / George H. Sakorafas -- Diagnostic strategies in acute appendicitis / Amato Antonio Stabile Ianora ... [et al.] -- Immunology of the appendix: effects of appendectomy / Juan Carlos Andreu-Ballester ... [et al.] -- Utilization of the Alvarado score to perform CT for acute appendicitis / Robert McKay, Roger Barrowman, Ellis Hospital -- Vermiform appendix: embryology, anatomy, and variations / Ahsan Rao, Irfan Ahmed -- Appendicitis during pregnancy: a serious disease and a diagnostic problem / L. Penninga, E.I. Penninga.
Subjects	Appendicitis. Appendectomy.
Notes	Includes bibliographical references and index.

Chinese medical obstetrics

LCCN	2006273082
Type of material	Book
Personal name	Flaws, Bob, 1946-
Main title	Chinese medical obstetrics / Bob Flaws.
Edition	1st ed.
Published/Created	Boulder, CO: Blue Poppy Press, c2005.
Description	x, 452 p.; 26 cm.
ISBN	1891845306
LC classification	RG524 .F565 2005
Related names	Flaws, Bob, 1946- Path of pregnancy.

Contents Nausea & vomiting of pregnancy -- Abdominal pain during pregnancy -- Ectopic pregnancy -- Spontaneous abortion -- Hydatidiform mole Habitual abortion -- Fetal growth disorders -- Missed abortion -- Edema during pregnancy -- Polyhydramnios -- Lower limb cramping & pain during pregnancy -- Lower limb varicose veins during pregnancy -- Pruritic urticarial papules & plaques of pregnancy -- Colds & flus during pregnancy -- Cough during pregnancy -- Hoarseness during pregnancy -- Diarrhea during pregnancy -- Dysentery during pregnancy -- Hemafecia during pregnancy -- Appendicitis during pregnancy -- Urinary tract infection during pregnancy -- Urinary retention during pregnancy -- Urinary incontinence during pregnancy -- Emotional dysphoria during pregnancy -- Heart palpitations during pregnancy -- Gestational diabetes -- Placenta previa -- Malposition of the fetus -- Dystocia -- Retained placenta -- Postpartum hemorrhage -- Postpartum infection -- Retention of lochia -- Postpartum lochiorrhea -- Postpartum dizziness -- Postpartum convulsions -- Postpartum uterine prolapse -- Postpartum aphonia -- Postpartum rib-side pain -- Postpartum low back pain -- Postpartum generalized body pain -- Postpartum headache -- Postpartum heart pain -- Postpartum cough -- Postpartum dyspnea and/or asthma -- Postpartum thirst -- Postpartum edema -- Postpartum hematuria -- Postpartum hemafecia -- Postpartum spontaneous perspiration & night sweats -- Postpartum constipation -- Postpartum diarrhea & dysentery -- Postpartum urinary stress incontinence -- Postpartum urinary

	retention -- Postpartum fatigue & exhaustion -- Postpartum insufficient lactation -- Postpartum areolar eczema -- Postpartum mastitis -- Postpartum weeping breasts -- Postpartum depression.
Subjects	Pregnancy--Complications--Treatment. Obstetrics. Medicine, Chinese. Pregnancy Complications--therapy. Obstetrics. Medicine, Chinese Traditional.
Notes	"This current edition is a combination of the previous Path of pregnancy, volumes 1 & 2, in a single volume."--Preface p. ix. T.p. verso lists book as the first edition of this title; preface lists it as the fourth edition of Path of pregnancy. Includes bibliographical references and indexes.

Cope's early diagnosis of the acute abdomen.

LCCN	2009013093
Type of material	Book
Personal name	Silen, William, 1927-
Main title	Cope's early diagnosis of the acute abdomen.
Edition	22nd ed. / revised by William Silen.
Published/Created	Oxford; New York: Oxford University Press, 2010.
Description	xiv, 299 p., [24] p. of plates: ill.; 21 cm.
ISBN	9780199730452 (pbk.: alk. paper) 0199730458 (pbk.: alk. paper)
LC classification	RD540 .S495 2010
Portion of title	Early diagnosis of the acute abdomen
Related names	Cope, Zachary, 1881-1974.

Contents	Principles of diagnosis in acute abdominal disease -- Method of diagnosis: the history -- Method of diagnosis: the examination of the patient -- Method of diagnosis: the grouping of symptoms and signs -- Laboratory and radiological tests -- Appendicitis -- The differential diagnosis of appendicitis -- Diverticulitis of the colon -- Perforation of a gastric or duodenal ulcer -- Acute pancreatitis -- Cholecystitis and othe causes of acute pain in the right upper quadrant of the abdomen -- Acute abdominal lesions arising in the left hypochondrium -- The colics -- Acute intestinal obstruction -- Intussusception and other causes of obstruction -- The early diagnosis of strangulated and obstructed hernias -- Acute abdominal symptoms due to vascular lesions -- Acute abdominal symptoms in women -- Early ectopic gestation -- Acute abdominal disease with genitourinary symptoms -- The diagnosis of acute peritonitis -- The early diagnosis of abdominal injuries -- The postoperative abdomen -- The acute abdomen in the tropics -- Diseases that may simulate the acute abdomen -- Acute abdominal pain in the immunocompromised patient -- Abdominal catastrophes when sensation is impaired.
Subjects	Acute abdomen--Diagnosis. Abdomen, Acute--diagnosis. Digestive System Diseases--diagnosis.
Notes	Includes index.

CT of the acute abdomen

LCCN	2011935932
Type of material	Book

Main title	CT of the acute abdomen / Patrice Taourel, editor; foreword by Albert L. Baert.
Published/Created	Heidelberg; New York: Springer, c2011.
Description	ix, 473 p.: ill. (some col.); 27 cm.
ISBN	9783540892311 (alk. paper) 3540892311 (alk. paper) 9783540892328 (e-ISBN) 354089232X (e-ISBN)
Publisher no.	12567478
LC classification	RC944 .C582 2011
Related names	Taourel, P. (Patrice)
Contents	Epidemiological data and clinical findings -- Epidemiology of acute abdominal pain in adults in the emergency department setting -- Epidemiology of abdominal trauma -- Elementary CT findings -- Key CT findings -- CT techniques -- Volume CT of acute abdomen: acquisition and reconstruction techniques -- CT diagnosis in non traumatic abdomen -- Acute liver disease -- Biliary emergencies -- Acute splenic disease -- Acute pancreatitis -- Acute appendicitis -- Ischemia (acute mesenteric ischemia and ischemic colitis) -- Diverticulitis -- Nonischemic colitis -- Acute gastritis and enteritis -- Bowel obstruction -- Bowel perforations -- Acute gastrointestinal bleeding -- Intra- and retroperitoneal hemorrhages -- Urological emergencies -- Gynecologic emergencies -- Acute diseases related to intra-abdominal fat in adults -- Acute disease of the abdominal wall -- Complications of abdominal surgery (abdominal, urologic and gynecologic emergencies) -- CT diagnosis in traumatic abdomen -- Abdominal trauma.

Subjects	Acute abdomen. Abdomen, Acute--radiography. Diagnosis, Differential. Digestive System Diseases--radiography. Tomography, X-Ray Computed--methods. Akutes Abdomen. Computertomographie.
Form/Genre	Aufsatzsammlung.
Notes	Includes bibliographical references and index.
Series	Medical radiology. Diagnostic imaging, 0942-5373 Medical radiology. 0942-5373

Doubting sex: inscriptions, bodies and selves in nineteenth-century hermaphrodite case histories

LCCN	2012406462
Type of material	Book
Personal name	Mak, Geertje.
Main title	Doubting sex: inscriptions, bodies and selves in nineteenth-century hermaphrodite case histories / Geerje Mak.
Published/Created	Manchester; New York: Manchester University Press, 2012.
Description	viii, 284 p.: ill.; 24 cm.
Links	Contributor biographical information http://www.loc.gov/catdir/enhancements/fy1304/2012406462-b.html Publisher description http://www.loc.gov/catdir/enhancements/fy1304/2012406462-d.html Table of contents only http://www.loc.gov/catdir/enhancements/fy1304/2012406462-t.html
ISBN	9780719086908 0719086906
LC classification	RC883 .M35 2012

Summary	"An adolescent girl is mocked when she takes a bath with her peers, because her genitals look like those of a boy. A couple visits a doctor asking to 'create more space' in the woman for intercourse. A doctor finds testicular tissue in a woman with appendicitis, and decides to keep his findings quiet. These are just a few of the three hundred European case histories of people whose sex was doubted during the long nineteenth century that Geertje Mak draws upon in her remarkable new book. How did people deal with such situations? How did they decide to which sex a person should belong? This groundbreaking analysis of clinical case histories shows how sex changed from an outward appearance inscribed in a social body to something to be found deep inside body and self. A fascinating, easy to follow, yet sophisticated argument addressing major issues of the history of body, sex, and self, this volume will fit advanced undergraduate courses, while challenging specialists."--Publisher's website.
Contents	Introduction -- Inscription. Secrecy and disclosure: politics of containment -- Early sex reassignments and the absence of a sex of self -- Herculine Barbin -- Body. How to get the semen to the neck of the womb -- Justine Jumas: conflicting body politics -- The dislodgement of the person -- Self. Sex assignment around 1900: from a legal to a clinical issue -- The turn inwards -- Scripting the self: N. O. Body's autobiography -- Conclusion.
Subjects	Intersexuality--History--19th century. Gender identity--History. Sex role--History.

	Disorders of Sex Development--history--Case Reports.
	Gender Identity--Case Reports.
	History, 19th Century--Case Reports.
	Role--Case Reports.
	Sexual Behavior--history--Case Reports.
Notes	Includes bibliographical references and index.

Emergency medicine evidence: the practice-changing studies

LCCN	2014017338
Type of material	Book
Uniform title	Emergency medicine (Antonsen)
Main title	Emergency medicine evidence: the practice-changing studies / Emily L. Aaronson, MD, Chief Resident, Harvard Affiliated Emergency, Medicine Residency, Department of Emergency Medicine, Brigham and Women's Hospital, Massachusetts, General Hospital, Boston, Massachusetts, Arjun K. Venkatesh, MD, MBA, MHS, Director, Quality and Safety Research and Strategy, Instructor, Department of Emergency Medicine, Scientist, Center for Outcomes Research and Evaluation, Yale University School of Medicine, New Haven, Connecticut, Erik L. Antonsen, MD, PhD, Assistant Professor of Medicine, Section of Emergency Medicine, Assistant Professor of Space Medicine, Center for Space Medicine, Baylor College of Medicine, Attending Physician, Ben Taub General Hospital, Houston, Texas; Special editors, Ron M. Walls, MD, FACEP, FRCPC, Jonathan N. Adler, MD, MS, FACEP, FAAEM.
Published/Produced	Philadelphia: Wolters Kluwer, [2015]
Description	xiii, 255 pages; 23 cm

ISBN	9781451192988 (pbk)
LC classification	RA645.5 .E45 2015
Related names	Antonsen, Erik, editor.
	Aaronson, Emily, editor.
	Venkatesh, Arjun, editor.
	Walls, Ron M., editor.
	Adler, Jonathan, editor.
Summary	"Ramp up your knowledge of the clinical trials and evidence that laid the groundwork for current emergency practice with Emergency Medicine: An Evidence Based Review. Brief, easy-to-read, and accessible, this time-saving quick-reference allows you to quickly familiarize yourself with the 100 most practice-changing clinical trials in emergency medicine. Features Master key information through one-page synopses of the 100 most-practicing changes clinical trials in emergency medicine. Explore landmark clinical trials in all areas of emergency medicine, including abdominal, airway, allergy, cardiology, endocrine, infectious disease, neurology, operations, orthopedics, pain, PE/DVT, psychiatry, pulmonary, toxicology, trauma, and ultrasound. Access crucial information you need to enter the world of evidence-based emergency medicine. Key findings in practical tips and commentary to improve your study Now with the print edition, enjoy the bundled interactive eBook edition, offering tablet, smartphone, or online access to: Complete content with enhanced navigation A powerful search that pulls results from content in the book, your notes, and even the Cross-linked pages, references, and more for easy Highlighting tool for easier reference of key

content throughout the Ability to take and share notes with friends and Quick reference tabbing to save your favorite content for future"--Provided by publisher.

Contents Machine generated contents note: Section 1: Abdominal Authors: Kathryn Hawk, Paulina Sergot. CT in the Diagnosis of Acute Appendicitis. Proton Pump Inhibitors in Bleeding Peptic Ulcer Disease. Somatostatin in Variceal Bleeding. Diagnostic Nasogastric Tubes in Hematemesis. Spontaneous Ureteral Stone Passage. Oral Ondansetron in Gastroenteritis. Oral vs. IV Rehydration in Children. Section 2: Airway Authors: Andrew Eyre, Brock Daniels, Anita Rohra. Non-Invasive Ventilation in Pulmonary Edema. End Tidal CO2 in Sedation. RSI in ED Training. Hemoglobin Desaturation after Succinylcholine. Laryngeal View Improvement in Laryngoscopy. Section 3: Allergy Authors: Christina Wilson, Brock Daniels. Cephalosporins in Penicillin Allergic Patients. Histamine Antagonists in Acute Allergic Reactions. Section 4: Cardiology Authors: Kenneth Bernard, Stephanie Burgos, Peter Pruitt, Harman Singh Gill, Joshua Keegan. TIMI risk score for ACS. Missed ACS in the ED. Acute MI without Chest Pain. Troponins in Chest Pain. Beta Blockers in AMI: The COMMIT Trial. Aspirin in AMI: The ISIS-2 Trial. Heparinizing Unstable Angina. Low Molecular Weight Heparin in Unstable Angina. PCI vs Lytics in Acute MI: The Gusto IIb Trial. PCI Timing in ACS. tPA in Acute MI: The Gusto Trial. Delaying Defibrillation for CPR in Cardiac Arrest. Therapeutic Hypothermia in Cardiac Arrest. CPR Quality in Out of Hospital Cardiac Arrest. Chest Compression only CPR. Amiodarone in Ventricular Fibrillation. Epinephrine in Cardiac Arrest. tPA in PEA Cardiac Arrest. Vasopressin vs. Epinephrine for Cardiac Arrest. Pill in the Pocket for Atrial Fibrillation. Rhythm Control in Atrial Fibrillation: The Affirm Trial. Risk of Stroke in Atrial Fibrillation Cardioversion. Section 5: Endocrine Authors: Daphne Morrison-Ponce. ABG vs. VBG in DKA. Bicarbonate in DKA. Section 6: Infectious Disease Authors: Kito Lord, Ashley Kockankek, Jennifer Carne. Early Goal Directed Therapy in Sepsis. The PORT Score in Pneumonia. Dexamethasone in Pediatric Bacterial Meningitis. Steroids in Adult meningitis. Doxycycline in Lyme disease. Intervention to Decrease Catheter-Related Bloodstream Infection. Delayed Antibiotic Treatment for Acute Otitis Media. Centor Criteria for Strep Throat. The Febrile Infant--3 Stories. Bacterial Infection in Febrile Infants with RSV. Section 7: Neurology Authors: David Yamane, Michael Billington. CT before Lumbar Puncture in meningitis. Steroids and Antivirals in Bell's Palsy. Prochlorperazine in Migraine. Metoclopramide in Migraine. tPA for Acute Ischemic Stroke: The NINDS Trial. Intra-arterial tPA in Acute Ischemic Stroke: The Proact II Study. Timing of tPA in Acute Ischemic Stroke. Expanded window for tPA in Stroke: The ECASS III Study. Determining Stroke Risk after TIA. Urgent Follow up for TIA: The EXPRESS Study. The Epley Maneuver for Vertigo. Risk of Seizure

Recurrence in Pediatrics. Section 8: Operations Authors: Christina Wilson, Ije Akunyili. Chest Pain Protocols in the ED. Stress Testing in the Emergency Department. Social Interventions for Alcohol Abuse. Section 9: Orthopedics Authors: Andrew Eyre. The Ottawa Knee Rules. The Ottawa Ankle Rules. Section 10: Pain Authors: Michael Billington. Morphine and the Clinical Abdominal Exam. Ketorolac vs Ibuprofen in Musculoskeletal Pain. Pain Management in the ED: The PEMI Study. Section 11: Venous Thromboembolism Authors: Fan Yang. Clinical Diagnosis of PE. The PERC Rule in PE. D-dimer in DVT and PE. VQ Scan in Acute PE: The PIOPED Trial. CT Imaging for Acute PE: The PIOPED II Trial. Section 12: Psychiatry Authors: Daphne Morrison-Ponce. Pharmaceutical Restraints for Psychotic Agitation. Section 13: Pulmonary Authors: Radhika Sundarajan, Joshua Keegan. Low Tidal Volume Ventilation in ARDS. Magnesium in Asthma. Dual bronchodilators in Asthma. Dexamethasone for Croup. Oral vs. IV Steroids in COPD. Antibiotics in COPD exacerbations. Pulse-Oximetry replaces Arterial Blood Gases. Section 14: Toxicology Authors: Sabrina Poon, Fan Yang, Spencer Greene, Silpa Gadiraju .Fomepizole in Ethylene Glycol Poisoning. Hyperbaric Oxygen in CO Poisoning. Acetaminophen Poisoning and Toxicity: The Rumack Mathew Nomogram. NAC in Acetaminophen Overdose. Hydroxocobalamin in Cyanide Poisoning. Digoxin Immune Fab in Digitalis Toxicity. Crotalidae Immune Fab in Snakebites. Section 15: Trauma Authors: Andrew

	Eyre, Eva Tovar, David Beversluis. Laparotomy in Abdominal Gun Shot Wounds. Permissive Hypotension in Trauma. Level One Trauma Center and Mortality. CT vs. X-Ray in Traumatic Cervical Spine Injury. The NEXUS Criteria and the Canadian C-Spine Rules. New Orleans Criteria and the Canadian Head CT Rules. ED Thoracotomies. Pediatric Head Trauma. Section 15: Ultrasound Authors: Christina Wilson, Dapnhe Morrison-Ponce. Point of Care Echo in Penetrating Cardiac Injury. Ultrasound in Central Line Placement. Ultrasound in Trauma. Ultrasound in Resuscitation Termination.
Subjects	Clinical Trials as Topic--Handbooks. Evidence-Based Emergency Medicine--Handbooks. Emergencies--Handbooks. Emergency Treatment--Handbooks.
Notes	Includes bibliographical references.

EMQs and MCQs for surgical finals

LCCN	2010039155
Type of material	Book
Main title	EMQs and MCQs for surgical finals / Hye-Chung Kwak ... [et al.].
Published/Created	Chichester, West Sussex, UK; Hoboken, NJ: Wiley-Blackwell, 2011.
Description	xvi, 332 p.: ill.; 22 cm.
ISBN	9781405199414 (pbk.: alk. paper) 1405199415 (pbk.: alk. paper)
LC classification	RD37.2 .E47 2011
Related names	Kwak, Hye-Chung.
Summary	"Revise and prepare for surgical finals with a wide range of questions and comprehensive answers

that test your knowledge and help you learn EMQs and MCQs for Surgery Finals is a unique study and revision resource for final examination practice covering all surgical sub-specialties. Each section of the book begins with a brief outline of the surgical topic followed by a range of clinically-based questions to test both knowledge and understanding. The final chapter contains a range of clinical cases that guide you through a real-life scenario on core knowledge tested earlier in the book. This is an essential resource for surgical finals preparation and will assist in providing a rapid refresher, testing understanding, indentifying areas of weaknesses and consolidating knowledge. All in all, a real must-have for any student sitting final surgical examinations.--Provided by publisher.

Contents Machine generated contents note: Essential skills in surgery -- 1 Pre-operative assessment -- Head and neck -- 2 Neurosurgery -- Head injury -- Extradural haematoma -- Subdural haematoma -- Subarachnoid haemorrhage -- Cerebrospinal fluid -- Hydrocephalus -- Cauda equine syndrome -- 3 Ear, nose and throat -- Epistaxis -- Earache -- Foreign bodies -- Tonsillitis -- Parotid swelling -- Thyroid swellings -- Thyroid cancer -- Thyroid gland and hyperparathyroidism -- Chest -- 4 Thorax -- Thoracic trauma -- Rib fracture -- Tension pneumothorax -- 5 Breast surgery -- Mastitis -- Fat necrosis -- Benign breast lumps -- Breast cancer -- Abdomen -- 6 Acute abdomen -- Overview -- Necrotizing fasciitis -- Sigmoid volvulus -- Shock -- ATLS -- 7 Foregut -- The oesophagus -- Dysphagia -- GORD -- Barrett's oesophagus -- Malignant oesophageal tumours -- Gastric cancer -- 8 Hepatobiliary disease -- Pancreatic cancer -- Liver abscess -- Benign hepatic tumours -- Hepatocellular carcinoma -- Cholangiocarcinoma -- Acute pancreatitis -- Chronic pancreatitis -- Pancreatic pseudocysts -- Gallstones -- 9 Spleen -- 10 Midgut -- Acute appendicitis -- Small bowel obstruction -- Meckel's diverticulum -- 11 Colorectal -- Diverticular disease -- Colorectal cancer -- Inflammatory bowel disease -- Lower gastrointestinal bleeding -- Haemorrhoids -- Fissure in-ano -- Fistula in-ano -- 12 Nutrition in surgical patients -- 13 Abdominal wall -- Inguinal Hernia -- Femoral Hernia -- Umbilical Hernia -- Incisional Hernia -- Pelvis -- 14 Gynaecology -- Ectopic Pregnancy -- Pelvic Inflammatory Disease -- Ovarian cyst -- 15 Urology -- Urinary tract infection -- Renal colic -- The prostate -- Prostate cancer -- Benign prostatic hypertrophy -- Renal cell carcinoma -- Bladder cancer -- Vascular -- 16 Vascular -- Abdominal aortic aneurysm -- Popliteal artery aneurysm -- Carotid artery disease -- Amputations -- Varicose veins -- Diabetic foot --; Peripheral vascular disease -- Acutely ischaemic limb -- Orthopaedic -- 17 Orthopaedic -- Brachial plexus injury -- Radial nerve injury -- Ulnar nerve palsy -- Carpal tunnel syndrome -- Shoulder dislocation -- Colles fracture -- Fractured neck of femur -- Osteoarthritis of knee -- Burns and plastics -- 18 Burns and plastics -- Useful procedures -- 19 Useful procedures -- Draining an abscess -- Urinary catheter insertion -- Examining stomas --

	20 Clinical scenarios -- Answers -- Appendix I: commonly used surgical instruments -- Appendix II: normal ranges for blood tests -- Appendix III: orthopaedic examination.
Subjects	Surgery--Examinations, questions, etc. Surgical Procedures, Operative--Examination Questions.
Notes	Includes bibliographical references.

Evidence-based imaging: improving the quality of imaging in patient care

LCCN	2011924338
Type of material	Book
Main title	Evidence-based imaging: improving the quality of imaging in patient care / L. Santiago Medina, C. Craig Blackmore, Kimberly E. Applegate, editors; foreword by Bruce J. Hillman.
Edition	Rev. ed.
Published/Created	New York: Springer, c2011.
Description	xx, 680 p.: ill. (some col.); 26 cm.
ISBN	9781441977762 (alk. paper) 1441977767 (alk. paper) 9781441977779 (e-ISBN) 1441977775 (e-ISBN)
LC classification	RC78.7.D53 E95 2011
Related names	Medina, L. Santiago. Blackmore, Christopher Craig. Applegate, Kimberly E.
Contents	pt. I. Principles, methodology, economics, and radiation risk. Principles of evidence-based imaging / L. Santiago Medina, C. Craig Blackmore, and Kimberly E. Applegate -- Critically assessing the literature: understanding error and bias / C. Craig Blackmore ... [et al.] --

Radiation risk from medical imaging: a special need to focus on children / Donald P. Frush and Kimberly E. Applegate -- The economic and regulatory impact of evidence-based medicine on radiology / David B. Larson -- pt. II. Oncologic imaging. Breast imaging / Laurie L. Fajardo, Wendie A. Berg, and Robert A. Smith -- Imaging of lung cancer / James G. Ravenel and Gerard A. Silvestri -- Imaging-based screening for colorectal cancer / James M. A. Slattery, Lucy E. Modahl, and Michael E. Zalis -- Imaging of brain cancer / Soonmee Cha -- Imaging in the evaluation of patients with prostate cancer / Jeffrey H. Newhouse -- pt. III. Neuroimaging. Neuroimaging in Alzheimer disease / Kejal Kantarci and Clifford R. Jack -- Neuroimaging in acute ischemic stroke / Katie D. Vo, Weili Lin, and Jin-Moo Lee -- Pediatric sickle cell disease and stroke / Jaroslaw Krejza ... [et al.] -- Neuroimaging for traumatic brain injury / Karen A. Tong ... [et al.] -- Neuroimaging of seizures / Byron Bernal and Nolan Altman -- Adults and children with headaches: evidence-based role of neuroimaging / L. Santiago Medina and Elza Vasconcellos -- Imaging evaluation of sinusitis: impact on health outcome / Yoshimi Anzai -- pt. IV. Musculoskeletal imaging. Imaging of acute hematogenous osteomyelitis and septic arthritis in children and adults / John Y. Kim and Diego Jaramillo -- Imaging for knee and shoulder problems / William Hollingworth, Adrian K. Dixon, and John R. Jenner -- Pediatric fractures of the ankle / Martin H. Reed and G. Brian Black -- Imaging of adults with low back pain in the primary care setting / Marla B. K. Sammer and Jeffrey G. Jarvik -- Imaging of the spine in victims of trauma / C. Craig Blackmore and Gregory David Avey -- Imaging of spine disorders in children: dysraphism and scoliosis / L. Santiago Medina ... [et al.] -- pt. V. Cardiovascular and chest imaging. Imaging of the solitary pulmonary nodule / Anil Kumar Attili and Ella A. Kazerooni -- Cardiac evaluation: the current status of outcomes-based imaging / Andrew J. Bierhals and Pamela K. Woodard -- Imaging in the evaluation of pulmonary embolism / Krishna Juluru and John Eng -- Aorta and peripheral vascular disease / Max P. Rosen -- Imaging of the cervical carotid artery for atherosclerotic stenosis / Alex M. Barrocas and Colin P. Derdeyn -- Blunt injuries to the thorax and abdomen / Frederick A. Mann -- pt. VI. Abdominal and pelvic imaging. Imaging of appendicitis in adult and pediatric patients / C. Craig Blackmore, Erin A. Cooke, and Gregory David Avey -- Imaging in non-appendiceal acute abdominal pain / C. Craig Blackmore and Gregory David Avey -- Intussusception in children: diagnostic imaging and treatment / Kimberly E. Applegate -- Imaging of infantile hypertrophic pyloric stenosis / Marta Hernanz-Schulman, Barry R. Berch, and Wallace W. Neblett III -- Imaging of biliary disorders: cholecystitis, bile duct obstruction, stones, and stricture / Jose C. Varghese, Brian C. Lucey, and Jorge A. Soto -- Hepatic disorders: colorectal cancer metastases, cirrhosis, and hepatocellular carcinoma / Brian C. Lucey, Jose C. Varghese, and Jorge A. Soto -- Imaging of inflammatory bowel disease in children / Sudha A. Anupindi ... [et al.] -- Imaging of nephrolithiasis and its complications in adults and children / Lynn Ansley Fordham ... [et al.] -- Urinary tract infection in infants and children / Carol E. Barnewolt ... [et al.] -- Current issues in gynecology: screening for ovarian cancer in the average risk population and diagnostic evaluation of postmenopausal bleeding / Ruth C. Carlos -- Imaging of female children and adolescents with abdominopelvic pain caused by gynecological pathologies / Stefan Puig -- Imaging of boys with an acute scrotum: differentiation of testicular torsion from other causes / Stefan Puig.

Subjects	Diagnostic imaging. Evidence-based medicine. Medical radiology. Nuclear medicine. Diagnostic Imaging. Evidence-Based Medicine.
Notes	Includes bibliographical references and index.

Feigin & Cherry's textbook of pediatric infectious diseases

LCCN	2008015063
Type of material	Book
Main title	Feigin & Cherry's textbook of pediatric infectious diseases / [edited by] Ralph D. Feigin ... [et al.].
Edition	6th ed.
Published/Created	Philadelphia, PA: Saunders/Elsevier, c2009.
Description	2 v. (xxxix, 3567, xciv p.): ill., maps; 29 cm.
ISBN	9781416040446 1416040447 9996036847 (vol. 1) 9789996036842 (vol. 1)

9996036901 (vol. 2)
9789996036903 (vol. 2)

LC classification RJ401 .T49 2009

Variant title Feigin and Cherry's textbook of pediatric infectious diseases

Portion of title Textbook of pediatric infectious diseases

Related titles Textbook of pediatric infectious diseases.

Related names Feigin, Ralph D., 1938-2008.

Contents V. 1: Molecular determinants of microbial pathogenesis -- Normal and impaired immunologic responses to infection -- Metabolic response of the host infections -- Interaction of infection and nutrition -- Fever: pathogenesis and treatment -- Indigenous flora -- Epidemiology of infectious diseases -- The common cold -- Infections of the oral cavity -- Pharyngitis (pharyngitis, tonsillitis, tonsillopharyngitis, and nasopharyngitis) -- Herpangina -- Pharyngoconjunctival fever -- Uvulitis -- Peritonsillar, retropharyngeal, and parapharyngeal abscesses -- Cervical lymphadenitis -- Parotitis -- Sinusitis -- Otitis externa -- Otitis media -- Mastoiditis -- Epiglottitis (supraglottitis) -- Croup (laryngitis, laryngotracheitis, spasmodic croup, laryngotracheobronchitis, bacterial tracheitis, and laryngotracheobroncho-pneumonitis) -- Acute bronchitis -- Chronic bronchitis -- Bronchiolitis and infectious asthma -- Nonbacterial pneumonia -- Bacterial pneumonias -- Children's interstitial lung disease and hypersensitivity pneumonitis -- Pleural effusions and empyema -- Lung abscess -- Cystic fibrosis -- Infective endocarditis -- Infectious pericarditis -- Myocarditis -- Acute rheumatic fever -- Mediastinitis -- Bacterial meningitis beyond the neonatal period -- Parameningeal infections -- Fungal meningitis -- Eosinophilic meningitis -- Aseptic meningitis and viral meningitis -- Encephalitis and meningoencephalitis -- Parainfectious and postinfectious disorders of the nervous system -- Urethritis -- Cystitis and pyelonephritis -- Renal abscess -- Prostatitis -- Genital infections -- Esophagitis -- Approach to patients with gastrointestinal tract infections and food poisoning -- Antibiotic-associated colitis -- Whipple disease -- Hepatitis -- Cholangitis and cholecystitis -- Pyogenic liver abscess -- Reye syndrome -- Appendicitis and pelvic abscess -- Pancreatitis -- Peritonitis and intra-abdominal abscess -- Retroperitoneal infections -- Osteomyelitis -- Septic arthritis -- Bacterial myositis and pyomyositis -- Cutaneous manifestations of systemic infections -- Roseola infantum (exanthem subitum) -- Bacterial skin infections --

Viral and fungal skin infections -- Ocular infectious diseases -- Bacteremia and septic shock -- Fever without source and fever of unknown origin -- Toxic shock syndrome -- Acute respiratory distress syndrome in children -- Viral infections of the fetus and neonate -- Chlamydia trachomatis infections in the neonate -- Mycoplasma and ureaplasma infections of the neonate -- Yeast and fungal infections of the fetus and neonate -- Congenital toxoplasmosis -- Perinatal bacterial diseases -- Primary immunodeficiencies -- Opportunistic infections in hematopoietic stem cell transplantation -- Infections in pediatric heart transplantation -- Infections of pediatric lung transplantation -- Opportunistic infections in liver and intestinal transplantation -- Opportunistic infections of kidney transplantation -- Infections related to prosthetic or artificial devices -- Infections related to craniofacial surgical procedures -- Infections in burn patients -- Kawasaki disease -- Chronic fatigue syndrome -- Nomenclature for aerobic and anaerobic bacteria -- Staphylococcus aureus infections (coagulase-positive staphlococci) -- Coagulase-negative staphylococcal infections -- Group A, group C, and group G beta-hemolytic streptococcal infections -- Group B streptococcal infections -- Enterococcal and viridans streptococcal infections -- Pneumococcal infections -- Miscellaneous gram-positive cocci -- Moraxella catarrhalis -- Meningococcal infections -- Gonococcal infections -- Diphtheria -- Anthrax -- Bacillus cereus -- Arcanobacterium haemolyticum -- Erysipelothrix rhusiopathiae -- Listeriosis -- Tuberculosis -- Other mycobacteria -- Leprosy and buruli ulcer: the major cutaneous mycobacterioses -- Nocardia -- Miscellaneous gram-positive bacilli -- Citrobacter -- Enterobacter -- Diarrhea-causing and dysentery-causing escherichia coli -- Klebsiella -- Morganella morganii -- Proteus -- Providencia -- Shigella -- Serratia -- Salmonella -- Plague (yersinia pestis) -- Other yersinia species -- Miscellaneous enterobacteria -- Aeromonas -- Pasteurella multocida -- Cholera -- Vibrio parahaemolyticus -- Vibrio vulnificus --

Miscellaneous non-enterobacteriaceae fermentative bacilli -- Acinetobacter -- Achromobacter (alcaligenes) -- Eikenella corrodens -- Elizabethkingia and chryseobacterium species -- Pseudomonas and related genera -- Stenotrophomonas (xanthomonas) maltophilia -- Actinobacillus actinomycetemcomitans -- Bartonellosis -- Tularemia -- Haemophilus influenzae -- Other haemophilus species (aphrophilus, ducreyi, haemolyticus, influenzae biogroup aegyptius, parahaemolyticus, and parainfluenzae) -- Hilicobacter pylori -- Kingella species -- Legionnaires' disease, pontiac fever, and related illnesses -- Brucellosis -- Pertussis and other bordetella infections -- Calymmatobacterium granulomatis -- Campylobacter jejuni -- Other campylobacter species -- V. 2: Streptobacillus moniliformis (rat-bite fever) -- Bartonella (cat-scratch disease) -- Borrelia (relapsing fever) -- Borrelia (lyme disease) -- Leptospirosis -- Spirillum minus (rat-bite fever) -- Syphilis -- Nonvenereal treponematoses -- Clostridial intoxication and infection -- Infant botulism -- Tetanus -- Actinomycosis -- Other anaerobic infections -- Classification and nomenclature of viruses -- Human parvovirus B_{19} -- Human bocaviruses -- Human polyomaviruses -- Human papillomaviruses -- Adenoviruses -- Hepatitis B and D viruses -- Herpes simplex viruses 1 and 2 -- Cytomegalovirus -- Epstein-Barr virus -- Human herpesviruses 6, 7, and 8 -- Varicella-zoster virus -- Smallpox (variola virus) -- Monkeypox and other poxviruses -- Mimiviruses -- Enteroviruses and parechoviruses -- Rhinoviruses -- Hepatitis A virus -- Caliciviruses -- Hepatitis E virus -- Reoviruses -- Orbiviruses, coltiviruses, and seadornaviruses -- Rotaviruses -- Rubella virus -- Alphaviruses -- Flaviviruses -- Hepatitis C virus -- Influenza viruses -- Parainfluenza viruses -- Measles virus -- Mumps virus -- Respiratory syncytial virus -- Human metapneumovirus -- Rabies virus -- Lymphocytic choriomeningitis virus infection -- Arenaviral hemorrhagic fevers -- Filoviral hemorrhagic fever: margurg and ebola virus fevers -- Coronaviruses and toroviruses, including severe acute respiratory syndrome -- Hantaviruses -- La crosse encephalitis and other California serogroup viruses -- Other bunyaviridae -- Human retroviruses -- Transmissible spongiform encephalopathies (Creutzfeldt-Jacob disease, Gerstmann-Sträussler-Scheinker disease, kuru, fetal familial insomnia, new variant Creutzefeldt-Jakob disease, sporadic fetal insomnia) -- Chlamydia infections -- Rickettsial and ehrlichial diseases -- Mycoplasma and ureaplasma infections -- Classification of fungi -- Aspergillus and aspergillosis -- Blastomycosis -- Candidiasis -- Coccidioidomycosis -- Paracoccidioidomycosis -- Cryptococcosis -- Histoplasmosis -- Sporotrichosis -- Zygomycosis -- Miscellaneous mycoses -- Classification and nomenclature of human parasites -- Amebiasis -- Blastocystis hominis infection -- Cryptosporidiosis -- Entamoeba coli infection -- Giardiasis -- Dientamoeba fragilis infections -- Trichomonas infections -- Balantidium coli infection --

Cyclosporiasis, isosporiasis, and microsporidiosis -- Babesiosis -- Malaria -- Leishmaniasis -- Trypanosomiasis -- Naegleria, acanthamoeba, and balamuthia -- Toxoplasmosis -- Pneumocystis pneumonia -- Parasitic nematode infections -- Cestodes -- Trematodes -- Schistosomiasis -- Arthropods -- International travel issues for children -- Infectious disease considerations in international adoptees and refugees -- Health care-associated infections -- Programs to prevent and control health-care associated infections -- Antibiotic resistance -- The pharmacokinetic-pharmacodynamic interfaceideterminants of anti-infective drug action and efficacy in pediatrics -- Antibacterial therapeutic agents -- Antimicrobial prophylaxis -- Outpatient intravenous antimicrobial therapy for serious infections -- Antiviral agents -- Antifungal agents -- Drugs for parasitic infections -- Immunomodulating agents -- Active immunizing agents -- Passive immunization -- Public health aspects of infectious disease control -- Infections in daycare environments -- Human bites -- Animal bites -- Bioterrorism -- Bacterial laboratory diagnosis -- Fungal laboratory analysis: specimen collection, direct detection, and culture -- Viral laboratory diagnosis -- Parasitic laboratory diagnosis -- Epidemiology and biostatistics.

Subjects Communicable diseases in children.
Communicable Diseases.
Child.
Pediatrics--methods.

Notes	Rev. ed. of: Textbook of pediatric infectious diseases / [edited by] Ralph D. Feigin ... [et al.]. 5th ed. c2004. "Expert consult"--Cover. Includes bibliographical references and index.

Gastrointestinal diseases and disorders sourcebook: basic consumer health information about the upper and lower gastrointestinal (GI) tract, including the esophagus, stomach, intestines, rectum, liver, and pancreas, with facts about gastroesophageal reflux disease, gastritis, appendicitis, ulcers, celiac disease, diverticulitis, irritable bowel syndrome, hemorrhoids, gallstones, and other diseases and disorders related to the digestive process; along with information about cancers of the gastrointestinal tract, food intolerances, and commonly used diagnostic and surgical procedures, statistics, a glossary, and resources for additional help and information.

LCCN	2015044229
Type of material	Book
Main title	Gastrointestinal diseases and disorders sourcebook: basic consumer health information about the upper and lower gastrointestinal (GI) tract, including the esophagus, stomach, intestines, rectum, liver, and pancreas, with facts about gastroesophageal reflux disease, gastritis, appendicitis, ulcers, celiac disease, diverticulitis, irritable bowel syndrome, hemorrhoids, gallstones, and other diseases and disorders related to the digestive process; along with information about cancers of the gastrointestinal tract, food intolerances, and commonly used diagnostic and surgical procedures, statistics, a glossary, and resources for additional help and information.
Edition	Third edition.

Published/Produced	Detroit, MI: Omnigraphics, Inc., [2016]
Description	xv, 731 pages: illustrations; 24 cm.
ISBN	9780780814578 (hardcover: alk. paper) 9780780814585 (ebook)
LC classification	RC806 .G37 2016
Related names	Omnigraphics, Inc.
Summary	"Provides basic consumer health information about the causes, symptoms, diagnosis, and treatment of digestive diseases and disorders affecting the esophagus, stomach intestines, gall bladder, liver and pancreas. It also includes facts about the effects of food intolerances, infections, and certain cancers. An index, glossary of related terms, and other resources are also provided"--Provided by publisher.
Subjects	Gastrointestinal system--Diseases--Popular works.
Notes	Includes bibliographical references and index.
Additional formats	Online version: Gastrointestinal diseases and disorders sourcebook Third edition. Detroit, MI: Omnigraphics, Inc., [2016] 9780780814585 (DLC) 2015044765
Series	Health reference series

Great Ormond Street handbook of paediatrics

LCCN	2017448853
Type of material	Book
Uniform title	Great Ormond Street colour handbook of paediatrics and child health.
Main title	Great Ormond Street handbook of paediatrics / edited by Stephan Strobel, MD, PhD, MRCP(Hon), FRCP, FRCPH, Honorary Professor of Paediatrics and Clinical Immunology, University College London

	Institute of Child Health, London, Lewis Spitz, MChB, PhD, MD(Hon), FRCS(Edin), FRCS(Eng), FAAP (Hon), FRCPCH, FACS(Hon), Emeritus Nuffield Professor of Paediatric Surgery, Great Ormond Street Hospital for Children NHS Foundation Trust and University College London Institute of Child Health, London, Stephen D. Marks, MD, MBChB, MSC, MRCP(UK), DCH, FRPCH, Consultant Paediatric Nephrologist, Great Ormond Street Hospital for Children NHS Foundation Trust and University College London Institute of Child Health, London.
Edition	Second edition.
Published/Produced	Boca Raton: CRC Press, Taylor & Francis Group, [2016]
Description	xxv, 710 pages: illustrations; 26 cm.
ISBN	9781482222791 (pbk.; alk. paper) 1482222795 (pbk.; alk. paper) (ePub ebook) (PDF ebook) (VitalBook ebook)
LC classification	RJ45 .G76 2016
Variant title	Handbook of paediatrics
Related names	Strobel, Stephan, author. Spitz, Lewis, author. Marks, Stephen D., author. Hospital for Sick Children (London, England)
Contents	Machine generated contents note: ch. 1 Emergency Medicine -- Introduction -- Upper airway obstruction -- Anaphylaxis -- Asthma -- Bronchiolitis -- Cardiac emergencies -- Cyanosis -- Cardiogenic pulmonary oedema -- Cardiogenic shock -- Arrhythmias -- Acute encephalopathic

illness -- Convulsive status epilepticus -- Other encephalopathic illness -- Diabetic ketoacidosis -- Acute respiratory distress syndrome -- Sepsis -- Trauma -- Traumatic brain injury -- The child with multiple injuries -- Bums -- Poisoning -- References/further reading -- ch. 2 Child Protection -- Introduction -- Types of abuse and neglect -- Paediatric assessment of a child with suspicion of maltreatment -- Physical abuse -- Neglect -- Sexual abuse -- Other considerations in child protection -- What to do when abuse is suspected -- Further reading -- ch. 3 Infectious Diseases -- Bacteria -- Diphtheria -- Tetanus -- Meningococcal infections -- Tuberculosis -- Tuberculous meningitis Non-tuberculous myeobacterial infections -- Cat-scratch disease -- Lyme disease -- Pyogenic liver abscess -- Staphylococcal toxic shock syndrome -- Tularaemia -- Viruses -- HIV infection and AIDS -- Congenital cytomegalovirus -- Infectious mononucleosis -- Measles -- Neonatal herpes simplex virus -- Varicella (chicken pox) -- Herpes zoster (shingles) -- Protozoa/fungi/tropical diseases/miscellaneous -- Congenital toxoplasmosis -- Cryptosporidiosis -- Cysticercosis (neurocysticcrcosis) -- Invasive aspergillosis -- Neonatal systemic candidiasis -- Malaria -- Schistosomiasis (urinary) -- Visceral leishmaniasis (Kala-azar) -- Kawasaki disease -- Further reading -- ch. 4 Respiratory Medicine -- Cystic fibrosis -- Chronic lung disease of prematurity -- Preschool wheeze -- Asthma -- Bronchiolitis -- Pneumonia -- Empyema -- Non-CF bronchiectasis -- Interstitial lung disease --

Pigmentary mosaicism -- Cafe-au-lait macules -- Congenital melanocytic naevi -- Blistering conditions -- Epidermolysis bullosa -- Immunobullous disorders -- Inflammatory conditions -- Eczema -- Morphoea (localized scleroderma) -- Psoriasis -- Lumps and bumps -- Anogenital warts -- Molluscum contagiosum -- Sebaceous naevus -- Aplasia cutis -- Other important conditions -- Acrodermatitis entcroparhica -- Incontinentia pigmenti -- Cutaneous mast cell disease Ichthyosis -- Linear epidermal naevi -- Ectodermal dysplasia -- Paediatric dermatological emergencies -- Stevens-Johnson syndrome and toxic epidermal necrolysis -- Staphylococcal scalded skin syndrome -- Collodion baby and harlequin ichthyosis -- Eczema herpeticum -- Generalised pustular psoriasis -- Malignant skin conditions -- Further reading -- ch. 7 Ophthalmology -- Anatomy of the eye -- Visual development -- Lids -- Ablepharon -- Cryptophthalmos -- Colohoma -- Fpicanthus -- Entropion -- Ectropion -- Symhlepharon -- Blepharitis -- Stye -- Molluscum contagiosum -- Capillary haemangioma -- Port wine stain -- Ptosis -- Lid retraction -- Preseptal cellulitis -- Lid lag -- The watering eye -- Cornea -- developmental disorders -- Microcornea -- Cornea plana -- Megalocornea -- Keratoconus -- Congenital corneal opacification -- Corneal dystrophies -- Posterior embryotoxon -- Corneal deposits -- Keratitis -- Conjunctiva -- Infection-related conjunctivitis Non infection-related conjunctivitis -- Conjunctival pigmentation -- Elevated conjunctival lesions -- Diffusely elevated conjunctival lesions -- Sclera -- Pigmentation of the sclera -- Scleral inflammation -- Developmental anomalies of the globc -- Nanophthalmos -- Simple microphthalmos -- Complex microphthalmos -- Anophthalmia -- Iris -- Congenital iris defects -- Acquired iris defects -- Changes in iris colour -- Leukaemia/lymphoma -- Heterochromia irides -- Pupil anomalies -- Leukoeoria -- Dyscoria -- Miosis -- Mydriasis -- Corectopia -- Anisocoria -- Lens anomalies -- Aphakia -- Abnormal shape -- Dislocated lens -- Lens opacity -- Retinal anomalies -- Haemorrhages -- Hard exudates -- Cotton wool spots -- Retinal ncovaseularisation -- Retinal vasculitis -- Fovcal hypoplasia -- Maculopathy -- Coloured macular lesions -- Pale retinal lesions -- Non inflammatory lesions -- Retinal detachment -- Folds in the fundus -- The optic disc Optic disc swelling -- Optic atrophy -- Small optic disc -- Large optic disc -- Large optic disc cup -- Optic disc vascular abnormalities -- Optic disc haemorrhages -- Lesions obscuring the optic disc -- The orbit -- Abnormalities of globe position -- Lacrimal gland enlargement -- Eye movement disorders -- Ocular deviation in primary gaze -- Anomalous eye movements -- Abnormal head positions -- Nystagmus -- Further reading -- ch. 8 Neurology -- Neurological examination: cranial nerves -- The eye -- Ptosis -- Myasthenia -- Disorders of eye movement -- Third nerve palsy -- Fourth nerve palsy -- Sixth nerve palsy -- Ophthalmoplegia -- Upward gaze palsy -- Lateral gaze palsy -- Facial palsy -- Lower motor neuron facial palsy -- Upper motor neuron facial palsy --

Lower cranial nerve abnormalities -- Motor system -- Pyramidal disorders -- Extrapyramidal disorders -- Wilson disease -- Sydenham chorea and other poststreptococcal movement disorders Anti-N-methyl-D-aspartate receptor (NMDAR) encephalitis -- Sandifer syndrome -- Segawa syndrome (DOPA-responsive dystonia) -- Ataxia -- Ataxia telangiectasia -- Friedreich ataxia -- Acute generalised weakness in a previously well child -- Guillain -- Barre syndrome -- Dermatomyositis -- Spinal cord disorders -- Hypotonia in infancy -- Myotonic dystrophy (DM1) -- Spinal muscular atrophy (SMA) type 1 (Werdnig -- Hoffman disease) -- Spinal muscular atrophy (SMA) type 2 and type 3 -- Chronic and progressive weakness in the older child -- Duchenne/Beeker muscular dystrophy -- Hereditary motor and sensory neuropathy (CMT) -- Cerebral palsy -- Spina bifida -- Headaches -- Migraine -- Psychogenic headaches -- Intracranial hypertension -- Idiopathic intracranial hypertension (̀benign' intracranial hypertension, pseudotumour cerebri) -- Macrocephaly -- Hydrocephalus -- Brain tumours -- Learning difficulties -- Epilepsy -- Neurological and cognitive deterioration Common conditions with neurological deterioration -- Coma and acute encephalopathies -- Stroke -- Further reading -- ch. 9 Gastroenterology -- Clinical presentation -- Acute gastroenteritis -- Faltering growth/failure to thrive -- Constipation -- Infantile colic -- Recurrent abdominal pain -- Toddler's diarrhoea -- Chronic intractable diarrhoea -- Chronic intestinal failure -- Gastrointestinal diagnoses --

Fabricated and induced illness -- Coeliac disease -- Food allergic enteropathy -- Autoimmune enteropathy -- Eosinophilic gastrointestinal disease -- Eosinophilic oesophagitis -- Eosinophilic enteropathy -- Eosinophilic disease of the colon (FDC) allergic colitis -- Classic inflammatory bowel disease -- Ulcerative colitis -- Crohn disease -- Lymphangiectasia -- Ulcers -- Gastric ulcer -- Duodenal ulcers -- Polyps -- Isolated inflammatory/juvenile polyp -- Juvenile polyposis syndrome -- Familial polyposis coli and Gardner syndrome Peutz -- Jegher syndrome -- Infections and infestations -- Bacterial enteric infections -- Feeding difficulties -- Gastro-oesophageal reflux -- Cyclical vomiting -- Intestinal pseudo-obstruction -- Short bowel syndrome -- Congenital and inherited disorders -- Congenital chloride diarrhoea -- Glucose -- glactose malabsorption -- Sucrose -- isomaltase deficiency -- Lactose malabsorption -- Pancreatic disease -- Cystic fibrosis -- Shwachman -- Bodian-Diamond syndrome -- Acute pancreatitis -- Chronic pancreatitis -- Liver disease -- Primary sclerosing cholangitis -- Chronic hepatitis -- Acute hepatitis -- Alagille syndrome -- Mineral disorders (deficiencies, high level poisoning) -- Zinc deficiency -- Iron deficiency -- Copper deficiency -- Copper excess: Wilson disease -- Selenium deficiency -- Vitamin deficiencies -- Scurvy, vitamin C/ascorbic acid deficiency -- Beriberi, vitamin B1/thiamin deficiency -- Pellagra, niacin deficiency Riboflavin/vitamin B2 deficiency -- Pyridoxine/vitamin B6 deficiency -- Cyanocobalamin/vitamin B12 deficiency --

Vitamin K/napthaquinune deficiency -- Retinol/vitamin A deficiency -- Tocopherol/vitamin E deficiency -- Vitamin D deficiency -- Further reading -- ch. 10 Renal Diseases -- Acute kidney injury -- Haemolytic uraemic syndrome -- Glomerulonephritis -- IgA vasculitis -- Nephrotic syndrome -- Chronic kidney disease -- Cystic kidney diseases -- Congenital anomalies of the kidney and urinary tract -- Vesicouicteric reflux -- Renovascular hypertension -- Renal Fanconi syndrome -- Further reading -- ch. 11 Haematology -- Non-Hodgkin lymphoma -- Haematological disorders and Down syndrome -- Transient myeloproliferative disorder -- Myeloid leukaemia and DS -- Acute lymphoblastic leukaemia and DS -- Acute promyelocytic leukaemia and thrombosis -- Congenital (monocytic and myelomonocytic) leukaemia -- Ophthalmic cxtramedullary leukaemic deposits Granulocytic sarcoma -- Hypopyon -- Severe aplastic anaemia -- Juvenile myelomonocytic leukaemia -- Paediatric myelodysplastic syndromes -- Fanconi anaemia -- Dyskeratosis Congenita and TINF2 mutations -- Hypereosinophilic syndrome and T(5;12) -- Acute febrile neutrophilic dermatosis -- Sweet syndrome -- Myelofibrosis and systemic lupus erythematosus -- Infant megaloblastic anaemia: transcobalamin II deficiency -- Congenital erythropoietic porphyria -- Kasabach -- Merritt syndrome -- Thrombocytopenia absent radius -- Bernard -- Soulier syndrome -- Von Willebrand disease -- Severe haemophilia A and B (classic haemophilia and Christmas disease) -- Red cell membrane abnormalities -- Hereditary elliptocytosis -- Hereditary spherocytosis -- Beta-thalassaemia major -- Sickle cell discasc -- Glucose-6 -- phosphate dehydrogenase deficiency -- Pyruvate kinase deficiency -- Further reading -- ch. 12 Oncology -- Introduction -- Renal tumours -- Liver tumours Langerhans cell histiocytosis -- Rhabdomyosarcoma, other soft tissue sarcomas and fibromatosis -- Rhabdomyosarcoma -- Other soft tissue sarcomas -- Neuroblastoma -- Very low- and low-risk neuroblastoma -- Intermediate-risk neuroblastoma -- High-risk neuroblastoma -- Retinoblastoma -- Paving sarcoma and peripheral primitive neuroectodermal tumour -- Osteosarcoma -- Extracranial malignant germ cell tumours -- Tumours of the central nervous system -- Ependymoma -- Medulloblastoma/PNET -- High-grade supratentorial glioma -- Brainstem glioma -- Low-grade astrocytoma -- Rare tumours -- Thyroid carcinoma -- Nasopharyngeal carcinoma -- Adrenocortical carcinoma -- Renal cell carcinoma -- Late effects of cancer treatment -- Further reading -- ch. 13 Endocrinology The short child -- Growth hormone deficiency/insufficiency -- Laron-type dwarfism -- Low birth weight syndrome -- Turner syndrome -- Prader -- Willi syndrome -- Skeletal dysplasias -- The tall child Marfan syndrome -- Pituitary gigantism -- Late puberty -- Klinefelter syndrome -- Early puberty -- Premature thelarche/thelarche variant or`benign' precocious puberty -- Gonadotrophin-dependent (central) precocious puberty -- McCune-Albright syndrome --

Polycystic ovarian disease -- Thyroid disorders -- Congenital hypothyroidism -- Acquired hypothyroidism -- Graves disease -- Adrenal disorders -- Primary adrenal insufficiency -- Gushing syndrome -- Ambiguous genitalia -- Congenital adrenal hyperplasia -- Disorders of glucose homeostasis -- Hyperinsulinism -- Type 1 diabetes mellitus -- Type 2 diabetes mellitus -- Monogenic diabetes -- Insulin resistance syndromes -- Other forms of diabetes -- Disorders of calcium metabolism -- Rickets -- Hypoparathyroidism/pseudohypoparathyroidism -- Hypercalcaemia -- Williams syndrome -- Further reading -- ch. 14 Metabolic Diseases -- Adrenoleukodystrophy -- Gaucher disease -- Hurler disease, MPS I Sanfilippo syndrome, MPS III -- Morquio syndrome, MPS IV -- Homocystinuria -- classical and secondary to remethylation disorders -- Wolman/cholesterol ester disease -- Fructose 1, 6-bisphosphatase deficiency -- Neuronal ceroid lipofusinoses -- Urea cycle disorders -- Galactosaemia -- Fatty acid oxidation defects -- Disorders of ketone body metabolism -- Tyrosinaemia -- Glycogen storage disease type I -- Peroxisomal biogenesis disorders -- Leigh syndrome -- Pyruvate dehydrogenase deficiency -- Pyruvate carboxylase deficiency -- Menke disease -- Phenylketonuria -- Biotin disorders -- Glutaric acidaemia type I -- GLUT 1 transporter deficiency -- Fabry disease -- Pompe disease -- Creatine deficiency disorders -- Methylmalonic and propionic acidaemia (MMA, PA) -- Neurotransmitter disorders (L-dopamine-responsive dystonia, tyrosine hydroxylase deficiency, pterin disorders) Sphingolipidosis disorders (Tay Sachs/Sandhoff/GM1/Niemann-Pick/metachromatic dystrophy/Krabbe) -- Congenital disorders of glycosylation -- Non-ketotic hyperglycinaemia (glycine encephalopathy) -- Smitrt -- Lemli -- Opitz syndrome -- Hypercholesterolaemia -- Further reading -- ch. 15 Genetics Introduction -- Common congenital malformations -- Chromosome disorders -- Chromosomes -- structural abnormalities and imbalance -- Roberrsonian translocation -- Chromosome mosaicism -- Trisomy 13 (Patau syndrome) -- Trisomy 18 (Edwards syndrome) -- Trisomy 21 (Down syndrome) -- Turner syndrome, 45, X and variants -- Williams syndrome -- 22q 11 deletion syndrome (DiGeorge syndrome) -- Single gene disorders -- Autosomal dominant inheritance -- Autosomal recessive inheritance -- X-linked inheritance -- Mitochondrial conditions and inheritance -- Genetic syndromes with cardiac malformation as a major feature -- The floppy baby -- Prader -- Willi syndrome Myotonic dystrophy (myotonic dystrophy type 1) -- Syndromes associated with features of a connective tissue disorder -- Children with severe developmental delay -- Angelman syndrome -- Rett syndrome -- Other common single gene disorders -- Duchenne muscular dystrophy -- Fragile X syndrome -- Neurofibromatosis type 1 -- Tuberous sclerosis -- Other rare recognisable syndromes -- Kabuki syndrome -- Rubinstein-Taybi syndrome -- Dc Lange syndrome -- Sotos syndrome -- Goldenhar syndrome (hemifacial microsomia) -- Vater/Vacteri association -- Bardet -- Biedl syndrome -- Beckwith-Wiedemann syndrome -- Silver -- Russell syndrome -- Albright hereditary osteodystrophy (pseudohypoparathyroidism type la) -- Further reading -- ch. 16 Immunology (Primary Immunodeficiency Syndromes) -- Background -- I.Combined immunodeficiencies -- Severe combined immunodeficiency -- Specific SCID sub-types -- Omenn syndrome (SCID variant) -- Adenosine deaminase (ADA) deficiency II.Other well-defined syndromes -- Wiskott -- Aldrich syndrome -- Cartilage hair hypoplasia -- Ataxia telangiectasia -- III.Thymic defects -- DiGeorge syndrome -- IV.Antibody deficiency syndromes -- Common variable immunodeficiency -- X-linked againmaglobulinaemia (Bruton disease) -- Hypogammaglobulinaemia with hyper-IgM (class-switch recombination) ch. 17 Rheumatology -- Introduction -- Juvenile idiopathic arthritis -- Systemic JIA -- Polyarticular onset: rheumatoid factor (RF)-negative JIA -- Polyarticular onset: RF-positive JIA -- Oligoarticular arthritis -- Enthesitis-related arthritis -- Psoriatic arthritis -- Arthritis associated with other chronic diseases -- Scleroderma -- Systemic sclerosis -- Localised scleroderma (morphoea) -- Juvenile dermatonmyositis -- Vasculitides -- Henoch Schonlein purpura (IgA vasculitis) -- Kawasaki disease -- Polyarteritis nodosa -- Anti-neutrophil cytoplasmic antibody-associated vasculitides -- Takayasu arteritis -- Systemic lupus erythematosus -- Overlap connective tissue disease -- Chronic recurrent multifocal osteomyelitis -- Periodic fever syndromes/auto inflammatory diseases -- Introduction -- Familial Mediterranean fewer -- Tumour necrosis factor receptor-associated periodic syndrome Mewalonatc kinase deficiency/hyperimmunoglobulin D periodic fever syndrome -- Cryopyrin-associated periodic syndrome -- Periodic fever, aphthous stomatitis, pharyngitis and adenitis -- Chronic pain syndrome -- Complex regional pain syndrome -- Joint hypermobility syndrome -- Further reading -- ch. 18 Neonatal and Gcncral Paediatric Surgery -- Oesophageal atresia -- Congenital diaphragmatic hernia -- Neonatal intestinal obstruction -- Meconium ileus -- Duodenal atresia -- Intestinal atresia -- Anorectal anomalies -- Hirschsprung disease -- Malrotation -- Duplications of the alimentary tract -- Necrotising enterocolitis -- Exomphalos -- Gastroschisis -- Umbilical hernia -- Umbilical anomalies -- Gastrointestinal haemorrhage -- Meckel diverticulum -- Pyloric stenosis -- Intussusception -- Sacrococcygeal teratoma -- Appendicitis -- Neck lesions -- Cystic hygroma -- Branchial sinus/cyst -- Preauricular sinus -- Sacral sinuses -- Dermoid cysts Thyroglossal cysts/fistulae -- Inguinal hernia -- Hydrocoele -- Undescended testis -- Torsion of the testis -- Phimosis -- Biliary atresia -- Cholcdochal cyst -- Vascular malformations -- Hemangioma -- Congenital vascular malformations -- Klippel -- Trenaunay syndrome -- Lymphoedcma -- Spina bifida -- Conjoined twins -- Farther reading -- ch. 19 Otorhinolaryngology -- Otitis media with effusion (glue ear') -- Acute otitis media -- Cholesteatoma -- Chronic suppurative otitis media -- Otitis externa -- Aural foreign bodies -- Congenital anomalies of the ear -- Preauricular sinus and abscess -- External ear anomalies -- Middle ear anomalies -- Inner ear anomalies -- Nasal polyps -- Rhinosinusitis -- Nasal glioma and nieningoencephalocoele -- Juvenile nasopharyngeal angiofibroma -- Nasal foreign bodies -- Choanal atresia -- Tonsillitis (acute, chronic and recurrent) -- Peritonsillar abscess (quinsy) -- Retropharyngeal abscess -- Obstructive sleep apnoea Drooling -- Laryngomalacia -- Recurrent respiratory papillomatosis -- Subglottic stenosis -- Laryngeal and tracheobronchial foreign bodies -- Branchial sinuses, fistulae and cysts -- Paediatric head and neck masses -- Thyroglossal duct cyst -- Oropharyngeal and oesophageal foreign bodies -- Further reading -- ch. 20 Plastic Surgery Cleft lip and alveolus +/- palate -- Cleft palate (isolated) -- Congenital melanocytic naevi -- Craniosynostosis -- Epidermolysis bullosa -- Extravasation -- Hemifacial microsomia -- Microtia and ear reconstruction -- Proteus syndrome -- Radial longitudinal deficiency -- Vascular anomalies -- Capillary malformations in later childhood -- Infantile haemangioma -- Acknowledgements -- References -- ch. 21 Orthopaedics and Fractures -- Normal variations of gait and posture -- Congenital and developmental abnormalities of the lower limb -- Postural abnormalities (the moulded baby) Congenital talipes equinovarus deformity (the club foot') -- Congenital vertical talus -- Developmental dysplasia of the hip -- Leg length discrepancies -- Fibula hemimelia -- Proximal femoral local deficiency -- Congcnital tibial deficiency -- Common congenital toe problems -- Other congenital/acquired lower limb problems -- Blount disease -- Congenital pseudarthrosis of the tibia -- Posteromedial tibial bow -- Pes eavus (the high arched foot) -- Classic causes of lower limb pain -- The child with a (painful) limp -- Bone and joint infection (osteomyelitis and septic arthritis) -- Transient synovitis vs. septic arthritis -- Lcgg -- Calve -- Pcrthcs disease (often called Perthes disease) -- Slipped upper femoral epiphysis -- Upper limb abnormalities -- Neonatal brachial plexopathy -- Torticollis -- Congenital upper limb anomalies -- Radial club hand -- Ulnar club hand -- Radioulnar synostosis -- Congenital dislocation of the radial head Other minor upper limb abnormalities -- Examples of generalised conditions affecting the musculoskeletal system -- Benign joint hypermobility syndrome -- Arthrogryposis -- Neuromuscular conditions with orthopaedic concerns -- Cerebral palsy -- Spina bifida -- The spine -- Congenital deformities -- Scoliosis -- Scheuermann disease (kyphosis) -- Spondylolisthesis -- Back pain -- Trauma -- Specific pacdiatric injuries -- Physcal injuries -- Pulled elbow -- Fractures around the elbow -- Lower limb injuries -- Pathological fractures -- Further reading -- ch. 22 Urology Congenital urine flow anomalies -- Hydronephrosis/Dilatation -- Pelviureteric junction anomaly (PUJA) -- Vesicoureteric junction anomaly (megaureter) -- Vesicoureteric reflux -- Posterior urethral valve -- Multi-cystic dysplastic kidney -- Renal agenesis, ectopia and fusion -- Duplex kidneys -- Incontinence -- Extrophy -- epispadias complex -- Neuropathic bladder -- Disorders of sex development Hypospadias -- Undescended testis -- Acute scrotum -- Urolithiasis -- Neoplasia -- Childhood renal tumours -- Wilms tumour (nephroblastoma) -- Genitourinary rhabdomyosarcoma -- Further reading -- ch. 23 Allergic Diseases -- Introduction: clarification of terms -- General diagnostic approaches for allergies and adverse reactions to foods -- Food allergy -- Food-induced anaphylaxis -- Asthma and allergic rhinitis: aspects related to food allergy -- Allergic asthma -- Atopic eczema -- Chronic urticaria -- Allergics/hypersensitivity to food additives -- Drug hypersensitivity and adverse reactions to drugs -- Management principles of cow's milk and other food allergies -- Further reading.

Subjects	Children--Diseases. Children--Health and hygiene. Pediatrics. Adolescent Health. Child Health. Infant Health. Children--Diseases. Children--Health and hygiene.
Form/Genre	Handbooks.
Notes	Preceded by The Great Ormond Street colour handbook of paediatrics and child health / Stephan Strobel [and others]. c2007. Includes bibliographical references and index.

Series	Pediatric diagnosis & management series Pediatric diagnosis and management.

Imaging of acute appendicitis in adults and children

LCCN	2011935930
Type of material	Book
Main title	Imaging of acute appendicitis in adults and children / Caroline Keyzer, Pierre Alain Gevenois, editors.
Published/Created	Berlin; New York: Springer, c2011.
Description	ix, 256 p.: ill. (some col.); 27 cm.
Links	Inhaltsverzeichnis. http://bvbr.bib-bvb.de:8991/F?func=service&doc_library=BVB01&doc_number=024522509&line_number=0001&func_code=DB_RECORDS&service_type=MEDIA B:DE-101 http://d-nb.info/1009480936/04 Inhaltsverzeichnis http://deposit.d-nb.de/cgi-bin/dokserv?id=3607960&prov=M&dok_var=1&dok_ext=htm Inhaltstext
ISBN	9783642178719 (hbk.: alk. paper) 3642178715 (hbk.: alk. paper) 9783642178726 (ebk.) 3642178723 (ebk.)
Publisher no.	Best.-Nr.: 80013501
LC classification	RD542 .I46 2011
Related names	Keyzer, Caroline. Gevenois, P. A. (Pierre Alain)
Subjects	Appendix (Anatomy)--Imaging. Appendicitis--Diagnosis. Appendicitis--therapy. Diagnostic Imaging--methods. Bildgebendes Verfahren. Blinddarmentzündung.

Form/Genre	Aufsatzsammlung.
Notes	Includes bibliographical references and index.
Series	Medical radiology. Diagnostic imaging, 0942-5373 Medical radiology.

Infectious pregnancy complications

LCCN	2009004979
Type of material	Book
Main title	Infectious pregnancy complications / Richard N. Canfield, editor.
Published/Created	New York: Nova Biomedical Books, c2009.
Description	xvi, 460 p.: ill. (some col.); 27 cm.
ISBN	9781607410386 (hardcover) 1607410389 (hardcover)
LC classification	RG578 .I545 2009
Related names	Canfield, Richard N.
Contents	Complications of infections in pregnancy / Dushyant Maharaj -- Infection related recurrent late abortions and preterm birth: early total cervix occlusion (ETCO) versus cerclage / Erich Saling and Monika Dräger -- Virulence of influenza virus on human fetal membrane tissues / Noboru Uchide and Hiroo Toyoda -- Serological response to rubella, herpes simplex 2 and cytomegalovirus in pregnant women with unexplained recurrent abortions / Maysaa El Sayed Zaki and Ahmmed Badawy -- Appendicitis during pregnancy: a serious disease and a diagnostic problem / L. Penninga and E.I. Penninga -- Mediastinal end subcutaneous emphysema as a complication of labor / Arkadiusz Praski ... [et al.] -- Program for the prevention of infection-related premature births: the role of the lactobacilli system and

vaginal pH / Erich Saling and Monika Dräger -- Challenges for the management of HIV-infected pregnant women in resource constrained settings / Stephen Mepham, Ruth Bland and Marie-Louise Newell -- Impact of materno-placental malaria, anaemia and HIV infection on perinatal outcome in Nigeria / C.J. Uneke ... [et al.] -- Toxoplasma gondii and pregnancy: priorities for diagnostics of congenital infection / Alessandra Sensini -- Screening for toxoplasma gondii infection in pregnancy in an urban area of northern Italy: management and problems / Massimo De Paschale and Pierangelo Clerici -- Rickettsioses in pregnancy / Maria Bitsori and Emmanouil Galanakis -- Infectious diseases of the urinary tract during pregnancy / Nándor Acs, Ferenc Bánhidy and Andrew E. Czeizel -- Dengue infection in pregnancy: pattern of hematological disturbance / Viroj Wiwanitkit -- Infectious diseases of the respiratory system during pregnancy / Andrew E. Czeizel, Nándor Acs and Ferenc Bánhidy -- Maternal outcomes in pregnancy with smallpox: epidemiologic investigations of case fatality, miscarriage and premature birth based on previous outbreaks / Hiroshi Nishiura -- Chicken pox infection in pregnancy / Viroj Wiwanitkit.

Subjects Communicable diseases in pregnancy.
Pregnancy Complications, Infectious.
Communicable Diseases--complications.
Genital Diseases, Female--complications.

Notes Includes bibliographical references and index.

Series Pregnancy and infants
Pregnancy and infants.

Introduction to emergency medicine

LCCN	2004023255
Type of material	Book
Main title	Introduction to emergency medicine / [edited by] Elizabeth L. Mitchell, Ron Medzon.
Published/Created	Philadelphia: Lippincott Williams & Willkins, c2005.
Description	xix, 708 p.: ill.; 26 cm.
Links	Table of contents http://www.loc.gov/catdir/toc/ecip051/2004023255.htm Publisher description http://www.loc.gov/catdir/enhancements/fy0712/2004023255-d.html
ISBN	078173200X
LC classification	RC86.7 .I586 2005
Related names	Mitchell, Elizabeth, 1957- Medzon, Ron.
Contents	History of emergency medicine / Benjamin Honigman -- Principles of resuscitation / Joseph H. Kahn -- Shock / Robert S. Chang -- Myocardial infarction / James Ford -- Pulmonary embolus / David Schindler -- Pneumothorax / Rishi Sikka -- Atypical chest pain / Rohit Gupta -- Congestive heart failure / Ron Medzon -- Asthma / Tipton -- Chronic obstructive pulmonary disease / Elizabeth Mitchell -- Pneumonia / Darcy Bittner -- Aortic dissection / Todd Thomsen -- Urolithiasis / Michael Filbin -- Pyelonephritis / Robert Murray -- Musculoskeletal disorder / Eric Legome -- Abdominal aortic aneurysm / Ami Dave -- Cholecystitis / Deborah Wong -- Appendicitis / Karen Casper -- Diverticulitis / Jeffrey Evans -- Gastrointestinal bleeding / David Peak, Diane Heller -- Bowel obstructions / Christopher Kabrhel -- Hyperemesis / Vicki Noble --

Gastroenteritis / M.W. Lai -- Abnormal vaginal bleeding in the nonpregnant patient / Laura Eliseo -- Complications of the first trimester pregnancy / Robert Dart -- Pelvic infections / Rebecca Steinberg -- Pelvic pain / Robert Dart -- Subarachnoid hemorrhage / Fred N. Jones -- Migraine / Thomas Perera -- Central nervous system infections / J. David Walsh -- Central nervous system neoplasms / Michelle Fischer -- Acute and chronic alcohol intoxication / Merle Carter, Edward Bernstein -- Metabolic disorders / Rob Lowenstein -- Seizure disorder / Joel Wasserman -- Psychiatric emergencies / Brendan Magauran -- Cerebrovascular accident / Ron Medzon -- Vertigo / Frank Carrano -- Syncope / Tara Director -- Neuromuscular weakness / Kerry McCabe -- Traveler's fever / Nanette Lugo -- Hiv and fever / Thea James -- Bacterial source of fever / Michael Snyder -- Fever of uncertain etiology / Brian Hession -- Prehospital emergency medical services systems / Alexander P. Isakov -- Disaster management / Kathyrn Brinsfield -- Hazardous materials / Sophia Dyer -- General approach to trauma / Simon Roy -- Musculoskeletal trauma / Elizabeth Mitchell -- Trauma during pregnancy / Robert P. Collins -- Burns / Mary H. Stewart -- Introduction to the poisoned patient / Sophia Dyer, Michelle Fischer -- Toxidromes / Edward W. Boyer -- Drugs of abuse / Michelle Fischer -- Cardiovascular medications overdose / Mark B. Mycyk -- Acetaminophen / Steven Wexler -- Salicylate overdose / Brook Beall -- Hyperthermia / Lamont Clay -- Hypothermia / J. Matthew Sholl -- Submersion injuries / Ted Curcio -- Electrical

	and lightning injuries / John Swanson -- Bites and stings / Robert L. Hood, Nicolas Jouriles -- Laboratory medicine / Peter W. Emblad -- Arterial blood gases / Peter W. Emblad, Corey Slovis -- Culturing fluids / Kevin G. Wheeler -- Pain management, analgesia, and sedation / Amy Kontrick -- Airway management / Keith Boniface -- Peripheral intravenous access / Patricia Maher Harrison -- Central catheter insertion / Kris Arnold -- Anesthesia: local anesthetic agents and regional blocks / Andreas Dewitz -- Wound care / Sangeeta Kaushik, Judith Linden -- Soft tissue infections / Jeff Schneider -- Lumbar puncture / Jonathan Wasserman -- Arthrocentesis / Lynn Dezelon, Katherine Manzon, Sandra Najarian -- Dislocations / Mark Bracken, Tri Tong -- Extremity splinting / William E. Baker.
Subjects	Emergency medicine. Emergency Medical Services--methods--Case Reports. Emergency Medicine--methods--Case Reports. Emergencies--Case Reports.
Notes	Includes bibliographical references and index.

Let's talk about when you have to have your appendix out

LCCN	2001000151
Type of material	Book
Personal name	Apel, Melanie Ann.
Main title	Let's talk about when you have to have your appendix out / Melanie Ann Apel.
Edition	1st ed.
Published/Created	New York, N.Y.: PowerKids Press, 2002.
Description	24 p.: col. ill.; 19 x 20 cm.
ISBN	0823958655 (lib. bdg.)

LC classification	RD542 .A64 2002
Subjects	Appendix (Anatomy)--Juvenile literature.
	Appendicitis--Juvenile literature.
	Appendectomy--Juvenile literature.
	Appendix (Anatomy)
	Appendicitis.
	Diseases.
	Appendectomy.
	Appendectomy--Child--Juvenile Literature.
Notes	Includes index.
Series	The let's talk library

Management of common problems in obstetrics and gynecology

LCCN	2010012059
Type of material	Book
Main title	Management of common problems in obstetrics and gynecology / edited by T. Murphy Goodwin ... [et al.].
Edition	5th ed.
Published/Created	Chichester, West Sussex; Hoboken, NJ: Wiley-Blackwell, 2010.
Description	xii, 548 p.: ill.; 29 cm.
Links	Contributor biographical information http://catdir.loc.gov/catdir/enhancements/fy1007/2010012059-b.html
	Publisher description http://catdir.loc.gov/catdir/enhancements/fy1007/2010012059-d.html
	Table of contents only http://catdir.loc.gov/catdir/enhancements/fy1007/2010012059-t.html
ISBN	9781405169165
	1405169168
LC classification	RG571 .M23 2010
Related names	Goodwin, T. Murphy.

Summary "For over 25 years, and through four prior editions, this book has espoused the "USC way" of managing clinical problems in obstetrics and gynecology. This fifth edition, again exclusively organized and written by the department faculty, fellows and residents, continues the tradition. Major milestones in our specialty, electronic fetal monitoring, ultrasound, colposcopy, and laparoscopy, formed an impressive panoply of techniques that were refined and firmly established in the last part of the previous century. Since the fourth edition was published 8 years ago, other advances have occurred, which will be addressed in this edition"--Provided by publisher.

Contents Cervical insufficiency and cerclage / Bhuvan Pathak, James A. McGregor and T. Murphy Goodwin -- Preterm premature rupture of the membranes / Paola Aghajanian -- Preterm labor: diagnosis and management / Joseph G. Ouzounian and T. Murphy Goodwin -- Post-term pregnancy / Patrick M. Mullin and David A. Miller -- Multiple gestations / Ramen H. Chmait -- Fetal growth restriction / Patrick M. Mullin and Marc H. Incerpi -- Rhesus disease and isoimmunization / Ramen H. Chmait -- Diagnosis and management of macrosomia / Joseph G. Ouzounian and T. Murphy Goodwin -- Labor induction / Patrick M. Mullin -- Abnormal labor / Emiliano Chavira and T. Murphy Goodwin -- Operative vaginal delivery / Marc H. Incerpi -- Shoulder dystocia / Joseph G. Ouzounian and T. Myrphy Goodwin -- Chorioamnionitis and postpartum endometritis / Marc H. Incerpi -- Vaginal birth after Cesarean / David A. MIller -- Placenta previa and abruptio placentae /

David A. Miller -- Placenta accreta / Richard H. Lee and David A. Miller -- Postpartum hemorrhage / Richard H. Lee -- Fetal death / Marc H. Incerpi and Ronna Jurow -- Assessing the obstetric role in the brain-damaged newborn / David A. Miller -- Lactation management / Brendan Grubbs -- Heart disease in pregnancy / Uri Elkayam and T. Murphy Goodwin -- Asthma during pregnancy / Martin N. Montoro -- Thyroid disease in pregnancy: hyperthyroidism / Martin N. Montoro and T. Myrphy Goodwin -- Thyroid disease in pregnancy: hyopthyroidism / Martin N. Montoro -- Seizure disorders and headaches in pregnancy / Laura Kalayjian -- Anemia and thrombocytopenia in pregnancy / Patrick M. Mullin and T. Murphy Goodwin -- Venous thromboembolism and inherited thrombophilias / Martin M. Montoro -- Systemic lupus erythematosus and the antiphospholipid syndrome / Martin N. Montoro and T. Murphy Goodwin -- Urinary tract infections in pregnancy: from symptomatic bacteriuria to pyelonephritis / Bhuvan Pathak -- Diabetes mellitus in pregnancy / Carolina Reyes -- Gastrointestinal disorders in pregnancy / Michael J. Fassett and Richard H. Lee -- Viral exposures during pregnancy / Alice M. Stek -- HIV in pregnancy / Alice M. Stek -- Trauma in pregnancy / Marc H. Incerpi -- Hypertension in pregnancy / David A. Miller -- Nausea and vomiting of pregnancy including hyperemesis gravidarum / T. Murphy Goodwin and Martin N. Montoro -- The acute abdomen during pregnancy: ovarian torsion, appendicitis / Marc H. Incerpi -- Mood and anxiety disorders /

Bruce Kovacs and Emily Dossett -- The older gravida / Bhuvan Pathak -- Obesity in pregnancy / Paola Aghajanian -- Teratogen exposure in pregnancy / Bruce Kovacs and Emiliano Chavira -- Electronic fetal monitoring: definitions and principles / David A. Miller -- Electronic fetal monitorinng: a systematic approach / David A. Miller -- Second- and third-trimester obstetric ultrasound / Guiliana S. Songster -- Prenatal screening for genetic disorders / Giuliana S. Songster -- Antepartum testing / David A. Miller -- Preconception counseling and reproductive life planning / Carolina Reyes -- Fetal lung maturation, the respiratory distress syndrome, and antenatal steroid therapy / Emiliano Chavira and T. Murphy Goodwin -- Fetal interventions / Ramen H. Chmait -- Vulvovaginitis / Aaron Epstein and Subir Roy -- Sexually transmitted diseases / Peyman Saadat and Subir Roy -- Genital herpes / Mario J. Pineda and Subir Roy -- Pelvic infection / Peyman Saadat and Subir Roy -- Prevention of postoperative surgical site gynecolgic infections / Uma Chandavarkar and Subir Roy -- Prepubertal vulvovaginitis / Jenny M. Jaque and Claire Templeman -- Dysmenorrhea / Uma Chandavarkar and Subir Roy -- Chronic pelvie pain / Judy Chen and Subir Roy -- Abnormal and dysfunctional bleeding / Marc J. Kalan -- Premenstrual syndrome / Sara Twogood and Jennifer Israel -- Adnexal masses / Judy Chen and Lynda D. Roman -- Ectopic pregnancy: diagnosis and management / Vanessa Sun and Donna Shoupe -- Endoscopic surgery / Allan S. Lichtman and Claire E. Templeman --

Postsurgical adhesion formation and prevention / Claire E. Templeman, Joseph D. Campeau and Gere S. diZerega -- Uterine leiomyomata / Brendan Grubbs and Robert Israel -- Breast disorders / Heather R. Macdonald -- Rectovaginal injiuries / Brendan Grubbs and Subir Roy -- Prepubertal vulvar lacerations and hematomas, labial adhesions, and prolapse of the urethra / Jenny M. Jaque and Claire E. Templeman -- Female sexual function and dysfunction / Lauren Rubal -- Endometriosis / Lauren Rubal and Robert Israel -- Urinary incontinence / John Klutke and Begüm Özel -- Urinary tract injuries / Micheline Wong and Begüm Özel -- Fistulae / Micheline Wong and Begüm Özel -- Pelvic organ prolapse / Micheline Wong and Begüm Özel -- Infections of the lower urinary tract / Christina Dancz and Begüm Özel -- Voiding dysfunction / Rebecca Urwitz-Lane and Begüm Özel -- Painful bladder syndrome/interstitial cystitis / Begüm Özel -- Urethral disorders / Rebecca Urwitz-Lane and Begüm Özel -- Anal incontinence / Ticaria Jackson and Begüm Özel -- Preinvasive disease of the lower genital tract / Amy D. Brockmeyer and Laila I. Muderspach -- Vulvar carcinoma / Merieme Klobocista and Laila I. Muderspach -- Vaginal carcinoma / Huyen Q. Pham -- Cervical cancer / Lynda D. Roman -- Endometrial hyperplasia: diagnosis and management / Huyen Q. Pham -- Endometrial carcinoma: evaluation and management / Melissa Moffitt and Laila I. Muderspach -- Ovarian carcinoma: management / Lynda D. Roman -- Special tumors of the ovary / Nannie A. Yessaian -- Trophoblastic neoplasia:

diagnosis and management / Annie A. Yessaian -- Precocious puberty / Marsha B. Baker and Mitchell E. Geffner -- Primary amenorrhea / Briana Rudick and Karine Chung -- Secondary amenorrhea / Briana Rudick and Richard J. Paulson -- Galactorrhea and hyperprolactinemia / Donna Shoupe -- Androgen excess and hirsutism / Rebecca Z. Sokol and Donna Shoupe -- Polycystic ovarian syndrome / Donna Shoupe -- Menopause / Lauren Rubal and Donna Shoupe -- Premature ovarian failure / Richard J. Paulson -- Human chorionic gonadotropin and the diagnosis of early pregnancy / Rene B. Allen ... [et al.] -- Work-up of infertility / Melanie Landay and Kristin A. Bendikson -- Induction of ovulation / Marsha B. Baker and Kristin A. Bendikson -- Male factor infertility / Rebecca Z. Sokol -- Uterovaginal anomalies: diagnosis and management / Donna Shoupe -- Tubal factor in infertility / Kristin A. Bendikson -- Unexplained infertility / Lauren Rubal and Richard J. Paulson -- Human in vitro fertilization and related assisted reproductive techniques / Richard J. Paulson -- Oocyte donation and third party parenting / Richard J. Paulson -- Fertility preservation and oocyte cryopreservation / Karine Chung and Richard J. Paulson -- Recurrent pregnancy loss / Melanie Landay and Richard J. Paulson -- Combination oral contraceptives, contraceptive patch and vaginal ring: indications, contraindications, formulations, monitoring / Daniel R. Mishell, Jr. -- Noncontraceptive effects of combination oral contraceptives / Daniel R. Mishell, Jr. -- Injectable and implantable contraception / Penina Segall-Gutierrez and Ian Tilley -- Intrauterine devices / Daniel R. Mishell, Jr. -- Barrier methods of contraception / De Shawn L. Taylor -- Fertility awareness family planning methods / Ian B. Tilley and Ronna Jurow -- Emergency contraception / Penina Segall-Gutierrez and Ian Tilley -- Medical abortifacients / De Shawn L. Taylor and Ronna Jurow -- Complications of surgical abortions / De Shawn L. Taylor and Ronna Jurow -- Tubal sterilization / Jessica Jocson and Robert Israel.

Subjects	Pregnancy--Complications. Generative organs, Female--Diseases. Genital Diseases, Female--therapy. Pregnancy Complications--therapy.
Notes	Includes bibliographical references and index.

My doctor, wine

LCCN	2003006939
Type of material	Book
Personal name	Derys, Gaston, 1875-
Uniform title	Mon docteur le vin. English
Main title	My doctor, wine / text by Gaston Derys; watercolors by Raoul Dufy; introduction by Paul Lukacs; translated by Benjamin Ivry .
Published/Created	New Haven: Yale University Press, 2003.
Description	xvi, 45 p.: ill. (chiefly col.); 24 cm.
Links	Table of contents http://www.loc.gov/catdir/toc/ecip041/2003006939.html
ISBN	0300101333 (cloth: alk. paper)
LC classification	RM256 .D4413 2003
Contents	Wine as food -- Vitamins and the radioactivity of wine -- Wine and childhood ailments -- Wine as a treatment for typhoid fever -- Wine for healthy

	kidneys -- Wine as a treatment for depression and anemia -- Wine as a treatment for appendicitis -- Wine as a treatment for diabetes -- Wine as a remedy for convalescents -- How wine affects the disposition -- How wine affects the morale -- Downfall of a lady teetotaler -- Wine as a treatment for obesity -- Wine maintains youth and beauty -- Wine is essential for writers -- Wine is necessary for artists -- Wine is essential for athletes -- Wine makes a fine figure of a man -- Long life thanks to wine
Subjects	Wine--Therapeutic use. Wine and wine making.
Notes	French text originally published in 1935.

Nursing care of the pediatric surgical patient

LCCN	2006025212
Type of material	Book
Main title	Nursing care of the pediatric surgical patient / editors, Nancy Tkacz Browne ... [et al.].
Edition	2nd ed.
Published/Created	Sudbury, Mass.: Jones and Bartlett Publishers, c2007.
Description	xxx, 531 p.: ill.; 29 cm.
Links	Table of contents only http://www.loc.gov/catdir/toc/ecip0618/2006025212.html
ISBN	0763740527 (casebound) 9780763740528 (casebound)
LC classification	RD137 .N87 2007
Related titles	Nursing care of the general pediatric surgical patient.
Related names	Browne, Nancy Tkacz.
Contents	Perioperative preparation of the child and family / Kathleen M. Leack -- Fluid and electrolyte

management of the pediatric surgical patient / Neil Ead -- Nutrition in the pediatric surgical patient / Amy W. Lamm and Kerin L. Worley -- Vascular access / Melanie A. Kenney -- Care of children with acute pain: operative, procedural, and traumatic / Wendy Lord Mackey and Renee C.B. Manworren -- Caring for the child with technology needs in the home / Kimberly Haus McIltrot -- Care and management of patients with tubes and drains / Lynne D. Farber -- Care of the child with an ostomy / Valerie E. Rogers -- Bowel management / Frances T. Gill and Linda J. Haga -- Common outpatient pediatric surgical procedures: inguinal and umbilical hernias, hydroceles, undescended testes, and circumcision / Mary Ellen Connolly and Carmel A. McComiskey -- Fetal surgery / Lori J. Howell, Susan R. Miesnik, and Kelli B.Young -- The surgical neonate / Kim Knoerlein ... [et al.] -- Necrotizing enterocolitis / Betty R. Kasson -- Common cysts / M. Elizabeth Foster -- Esophageal defects / Danuta E. Nowicki -- Congenital lung malformations / Teri Coha -- Common thoracic problems / Frances T. Gill -- Abdominal wall defects / Beth T. Zimmermann -- Intestinal atresias, duplications, and meconium ileus / Judith J. Stellar and Kelli B. Young -- Hirschsprung's disease / Melinda Klar -- Anorectal malformations in children / Kathleen O'Connor Guardino -- Hypertrophic pyloric stenosis / Kimberly O'Dowd -- Gastroesophageal reflux disease: recognition and management / Frances N. Price -- Malrotation and volvulus / Jeannette A. Diana-Zerpa and Tina J. Shapiro-

	Stolar -- Intussusception / Lynn E. Fagerman and Lynne D. Farber -- Appendicitis / Cynthia A. Bishop and Mary Ellen Carter -- Splenectomy, cholecystectomy, and meckel's diverticulum / Mary E. Otten and Marilyn Miller Stoops -- Biliary atresia and choledochal cyst / Laura M. Flanigan -- Solid tumors / Laura E. San Miguel -- Pediatric abdominal organ transplants / Kathleen Falkenstein, Kurt Freer, Michael J. Kinney, and Caroline Braas -- An adolescent bariatric weight management program / Nancy Tkacz Browne and Beverly Bynum Haynes -- Pediatric trauma / Pam Pieper -- Burn care of children / Robin Moushey, Lisa Meadows, and Jennifer Seigel -- Wound management in neonates, children, and adolescents / Valerie E. Rogers.
Subjects	Children--Surgery--Nursing. Pediatric Nursing. Perioperative Nursing. Child. Infant.
Notes	Rev. ed. of: Nursing care of the general pediatric surgical patient / edited by Barbara V. Wise ... [et al.]. 2000. Includes bibliographical references and index.

Oliver Bean, doctors aren't mean!

LCCN	2010284448
Type of material	Book
Personal name	Bacon, Joy.
Main title	Oliver Bean, doctors aren't mean! / written by Joy Bacon; illustrated by Edward J. Russell Elementary School students, Pine Bush, New York.

Edition	1st ed.
Published/Created	Warwick, N.Y.: Moo Press, c2007.
Description	1 v. (unpaged): col. ill.; 16 x 24 cm.
ISBN	9780979237119 (pbk.) 0979237114 (pbk.)
LC classification	PZ8.3.B134 Oi 2007
Variant title	Oliver Bean, doctors are not mean!
Related names	Edward J. Russell Elementary School (Pine Bush, N.Y.)
Summary	When Oliver Bean feels a pain in his side, he is apprehensive about visiting his doctor, but once he gets to the hospital, he finds out that the doctors and nurses are nicer than he had imagined.
Subjects	Bean, Oliver (Fictitious character)--Juvenile fiction. Doctors--Juvenile fiction. Hospitals--Juvenile fiction. Stories in rhyme--Juvenile fiction. Medical care--Fiction. Physicians--Fiction. Hospitals--Fiction. Appendicitis--Fiction. Stories in rhyme. Children's art. Medical care--Fiction. Physicians--Fiction. Hospitals--Fiction. Appendicitis--Fiction. Stories in rhyme. Children's art.

Pain sourcebook: basic consumer health information about specific forms of acute and chronic pain, including muscle and skeletal pain, nerve pain, cancer pain, and disorders characterized by pain, such as fibromyalgia ...

LCCN	2002066221
Type of material	Book
Main title	Pain sourcebook: basic consumer health information about specific forms of acute and chronic pain, including muscle and skeletal pain, nerve pain, cancer pain, and disorders characterized by pain, such as fibromyalgia ... / edited by Karen Bellenir.
Edition	2nd ed.
Published/Created	Detroit: Omnigraphics, c2002.
Description	xiii, 670 p.: ill.; 24 cm.
Links	Table of contents http://www.loc.gov/catdir/toc/fy031/2002066221.html Book review (E-STREAMS) http://www.e-streams.com/es0512/es0512_2211.html
ISBN	0780806123 (hbk.: alk. paper)
LC classification	RB127 .P346 2002
Related names	Bellenir, Karen.
Contents	Machine generated contents note: Part I: Pain -- Chapter 1-Pain: Theories, Treatments, and Hope 3 -- Chapter 2-What We Know about Pain 17 -- Chapter 3-Chronic Nonmalignant Pain 27 -- Chapter 4-How Is Nerve Pain Different from Physical Pain? 31 -- Chapter 5-Gender and Pain 39 -- Chapter 6-Pain in Infants 49 -- Chapter 7-Children with Pain 53 -- Chapter 8-Pain in the Elderly 57 -- Chapter 9-Roadblocks to Pain Relief 65 --Part II: Types of Pain and Disorders Characterized by Pain -- Chapter 10-Appendicitis 75 -- Chapter 11-Arthritis 77 -- Chapter 12-Back

Pain 87 -- Chapter 13-Cancer Pain 93 -- Chapter 14-Carpal Tunnel Syndrome 109 -- Chapter 15-Central Pain Syndrome 113 -- Chapter 16-Chest Pain 125 -- Chapter 17-Complex Regional Pain Syndrome 135 -- Chapter 18-Earache (Otitis Media) 141 -- Chapter 19-Fibromyalgia 149 -- Chapter 20-Gout 161 -- Chapter 21-Headache 169 -- Chapter 22-Heartburn 187 -- Chapter 23-Interstitial Cystitis 197 -- Chapter 24-Kidney Stones 205 -- Chapter 25-Myofascial Pain Syndrome 221 -- Chapter 26-Neck Pain 223 -- Chapter 27-Occipital Neuralgia 231 -- Chapter 28-Paresthesia 233 -- Chapter 29-Pelvic Pain 235 -- Chapter 30-Phantom Pain 249 -- Chapter 31-Pinched Nerves 253 -- Chapter 32-Polymyalgia Rheumatica and Giant Cell Arteritis 255 -- Chapter 33-Polyneuropathy 261 -- Chapter 34-Reflex Sympathetic Dystrophy Syndrome. 265 -- Chapter 35-Sciatica 271 -- Chapter 36-Sexual Pain (Dyspareunia) 273 -- Chapter 37-Shingles 281 -- Chapter 38-Shoulder Pain 289 -- Chapter 39-Temporomandibular Disorders (TMD) 303 -- Chapter 40-Thoracic Outlet Syndrome 309 -- Chapter 41-Tooth Pain 311 -- Chapter 42-Trigeminal Neuralgia 315 -- Chapter 43-Vulvar Pain (Vulvodynia) 319 --Part III: Pain Management -- Chapter 44-Principles of Pain Management 327 -- Chapter 45-Answers for Pain Patients 335 -- Chapter 46-Managing Pain in Palliative Care 339 -- Chapter 47-Pain Treatments: An Overview 351 -- Chapter 48-Ways to Take Pain Medicine 357 -- Chapter 49-Tolerance, Physical Dependence, and Addiction 361 -- Chapter 50-Risks of Prescription Drug

Abuse 365 -- Chapter 51-Opioids for People with Severe Pain 373 -- Chapter 52-Patient Controlled Analgesia (PCA) 379 -- Chapter 53-OxyContin 383 -- Chapter 54-Actiq for Breakthrough Cancer Pain 387 -- Chapter 55-Vioxx for Osteoarthritis and Menstrual Pain 389 -- Chapter 56-New Arthritis Drugs 391 -- Chapter 57-Non-Drug Adjuncts to Pain Medication 397 -- Chapter 58-Acupuncture 401 -- Chapter 59-Clinical Psychophysiology, Biofeedback, -- and Neurofeedback 425 -- Chapter 60-Hypnosis, Relaxation, and Massage Therapies 433 -- Chapter 61-National Institutes of Health Endorses -- Alternative Therapies for Chronic Pain -- and Insomnia 439 --Part IV: Living with Pain -- Chapter 62-Action Guide for People with Pain 445 -- Chapter 63-Keeping a Pain Diary 453 -- Chapter 64-Alcohol-Medication Interactions 455 -- Chapter 65-Painkillers and the Kidney (Analgesic Nephropathy) 465 -- Chapter 66-Pain Relievers and Peptic Ulcers 467 -- Chapter 67-Harmful Effects of Medicines on the Digestive System 469 -- Chapter 68-Chronic Pain and Depression 479 -- Chapter 69-Anger: Helpful or Harmful? 483 -- Chapter 70-Anxiety and Its Effect on Pain Perception 487 -- Chapter 71-Interpersonal Relationships and Pain 491 -- Chapter 72-Sexual Expression and Chronic Pain 495 -- Chapter 73-Sleep and Chronic Pain 499 -- Chapter 74-Chronic Pain: Financial Issues 505 -- Chapter 75-Physical Pain and Suicide 509 --Part V: Pain Research -- Chapter 76-The Need for Pain Research 519 -- Chapter 77-Complementary and Alternative Medicine: -- Research Challenges 523

Subjects	Pain--Popular works.
Notes	Includes bibliographical references and index.
Series	Health reference series Health reference series (Unnumbered)

Patient safety: investigating and reporting serious clinical incidents

LCCN	2016026643
Type of material	Book
Personal name	Kelsey, Russell, author.
Main title	Patient safety: investigating and reporting serious clinical incidents / Russell Kelsey.
Published/Produced	Boca Raton: CRC Press, [2017]
ISBN	9781498781169 (pbk.: alk. paper)
LC classification	R729.8
Contents	Introduction: why do we still miss appendicitis? -- RCA: background and context -- How do we recognise serious clinical incidents? -- Recognising serious incidents using the SIRT: case studies -- A culture of complaint: openness, candour, and blame -- Root cause analysis: what happened?: the evidence -- Root cause analysis: what happened?: care and service delivery problems -- Root cause analysis: understanding why -- Understanding why: system factors -- Human factors part 1: the key to enhanced learning -- Human factors part 2: situational awareness and high pressure environments -- Root cause -- Learning and recommendations -- Solutions design and changing cultures -- Writing reports.
Subjects	Patient Safety Root Cause Analysis--methods Safety Management--methods Medical Errors--prevention & control

Mandatory Reporting

Prenatal and postnatal care: a woman-centered approach

LCCN	2013024996
Type of material	Book
Main title	Prenatal and postnatal care: a woman-centered approach / edited by Robin G. Jordan, Julie Marfell, Janet Engstrom, Cindy Farley.
Published/Produced	Ames, Iowa: Wiley-Blackwell, 2014.
Description	xxviii, 668 pages: illustrations; 28 cm.
ISBN	9780470960479 (paper: alk. paper) 0470960477 (paper: alk. paper)
LC classification	RJ254 .P726 2014
Related names	Jordan, Robin G., 1954- editor of compilation. Marfell, Julie, editor of compilation. Engstrom, Janet, editor of compilation. Farley, Cindy L., editor of compilation.
Partial contents	pt. I. Physiological foundations of prenatal and postnatal care. 1. Reproductive tract structure and function / Patricia W. Caudle: Anatomy of the female reproductive system; Menstrual cycle physiology -- 2. Conception, implantation, and embryonic and fetal development / Patricia W. Caudle: Conception and implantation; The placenta; The embryo; The fetus -- 3. Maternal physiological alterations during pregnancy / Patricia W. Caudle: Hematologic system adaptations; Cardiovascular changes; Respiratory adaptations; Renal adaptations; Gastrointestinal adaptations; Metabolic changes; Skin changes; Hair and nail changes; Immunologic changes; Neurological and sensory changes; Musculoskeletal adaptations; Endocrine changes -- pt. II. Preconception and prenatal care. 4.

Preconception care / Victoria L. Baker: Challenges to providing preconception care; Benefits of preconception care; Evidence supporting preconception care; Content of preconception care -- 5. Prenatal care: goals, structure, and components / Carrie S. Klima: A brief history of prenatal care; Current goals for prenatal care; Structure of prenatal care; A new model of prenatal care: Centering Pregnancy; Components of prenatal care -- 6. Nutrition during pregnancy / Robin G. Jordan and Julie A. Paul: Understanding food units; Size of food servings; Prenatal nutrition and health outcomes; Nutritional needs in pregnancy; Macronutrients: total energy; Macronutrients: fats; Macronutrients: carbohydrates; Micronutrients; Weight gain in pregnancy; Food safety during pregnancy; Factors influencing nutritional intake; Making a nutritional assessment; Counseling for optimal prenatal nutrition; Special issues in nutrition -- 7. Pregnancy diagnosis and gestational age assessment / Janet L. Engstrom and Joyce D. Cappiello: Early pregnancy diagnosis and gestational age assessment; Pregnancy diagnosis; Gestational age assessment; Counseling for pregnancy diagnosis -- 8. Risk assessment and risk management in prenatal care / Robin G. Jordan: Process and purpose of risk assessment; Benefits of risk assessment; Limitations; Disadvantages of risk assessment and risk management; Misapplication of risk assessment and risk management; Perspective of risk and risk screening; Explaining risk to women; Potential problems of risk miscommunication; Informed consent -- 9. Prenatal genetic counseling, screening, and diagnosis / Robin G. Hordan and Janet L. Engstrom: Family history and risk evaluation; Genetic screening procedures offered to all pregnant women; Ethnicity-based genetic screening; Diagnostic prenatal genetic testing procedures; Developments in genetic testing options; Scope of practice considerations; Ethical considerations in genetic screening; Communicating about genetic testing and risk during prenatal care; Psychosocial effects in genetic testing; Perspective on genetic counseling during prenatal care -- 10. Assessment of fetal well-being / Jenifer Fahey: Physiological principles and indications for antenatal fetal surveillance; Scope of practice considerations; Antenatal fetal testing methods; Education and counseling; Cultural, personal, and family considerations; Health disparities and vulnerable populations; Legal and liability issues -- 11. Common discomforts of pregnancy / Robin G. Jordan: Back pain and pelvic girdle pain; Bleeding gums; Breast tenderness; Carpal tunnel syndrome (CTS); Cervical pain; Constipation; Dizziness/syncope; Edema; Emotional changes; Fatigue; Flatulence; Headache; Heartburn; Heart palpitations; Hemorrhoids; Increased warmth and perspiration; Leukorrhea; Leg cramps; Nasal congestion and epistaxis; Nausea and/or vomiting during pregnancy; Ptyalism; Restless leg syndrome (RLS); Round ligament pain; Shortness of breath; Skin changes; Hair and nail changes; Sleep disturbances; Supine hypotension syndrome (SHS); Urinary frequency; Urinary incontinence; Varicosities (legs/vulva); Visual changes -- 12. Medication use during pregnancy / Mary C. Brucker and Tekoa L. King: Pharmacologic terms; Types of pharmaceutical agents; Prescriptive authority; Governmental oversight of pharmaceutical agents; The prescription: essential components; Drugs and pregnancy; Teratology; Pharmacokinetics in pregnancy; Rational use of drugs in pregnancy -- 13. Substance use during pregnancy / Daisy J. Goodman, Alane B. O'Connor, and Kelley A. Bowden: Risks of perinatal substance abuse; Prevalence of prenatal substance abuse; Definitions; Historical approaches to maternal substance use; Harm reduction approach to prenatal substance abuse Position statements on prenatal substance use; Comorbid conditions and prenatal substance use; Commonly abused substances and pregnancy implications; Screening for prenatal substance abuse; Brief intervention and treatment; Smoking cessation during pregnancy; Care of pregnant women with substance use disorders; Referral to treatment; Opioid replacement therapy in pregnancy; Communication and coordination of care; Neonatal abstinence syndrome; Postpartum care; Cultural considerations; Personal and family considerations; Scope of practice considerations -- 14. Social issues in pregnancy / Nena R. Harris: Poverty; Incarceration; Intimate partner violence during pregnancy; Pregnancy and a history of childhood sexual abuse -- 15. Exercise, recreational and occupational issues, and intimate relationships in pregnancy / Meghan Garland:

Exercise in pregnancy; Environmental exposures in pregnancy; Sexuality in pregnancy; Working during pregnancy -- 16. Psychosocial adaptations in pregnancy / Cindy L. Farley: Maternal attachment and adaptation; Sibling adaptation and attachment; Partner adaptation and attachment; Body image; Childbirth confidence -- 17. Health education during pregnancy / Lisa Hanson, Leona VandeVusse, and Kathryn Shisler Harrod: Sources and quality of consumer childbirth education; Prenatal visit approach to individual childbirth education; Class education and group prenatal care; Developmental considerations in prenatal health education; Issues integral to prenatal education; Prioritizing prenatal education needs; Trimester-based approaches to prenatal education; Cultural considerations; Health disparities and vulnerable populations; Documentation of teaching -- 18. Assessment and care at the onset of labor / Amy Marowitz: Determining the onset of labor; Timing of admission to the birth setting; What is "false labor"?; Determining active labor; Anticipatory guidance during the prenatal period; Data collection; Plan of care; Sleep and rest; Coping strategies and comfort measures for early labor; Ambulation in early labor -- pt. III. Common complications of pregnancy. 19. Bleeding during pregnancy / Robin G. Jordan: Bleeding during the first half of pregnancy; Evaluation; Subchorionic hemorrhage or hematoma; Leiomyomas; Spontaneous pregnancy loss; Ectopic pregnancy; Gestational trophoblastic disease; Early pregnancy bleeding and scope of practice considerations; Bleeding during the second half of pregnancy; Placenta previa; Placental abruption; Diagnosis and management of bleeding in the second half of pregnancy; Scope of practice considerations in later pregnancy bleeding; Family considerations in later pregnancy -- 20. Amniotic fluid and fetal growth disorders / Victoria H. Burslem and Cindy L. Farley: Amniotic fluid dynamics; Normal placentation and fetal development; Amniotic fluid disorders; Fetal growth disorders; Intrauterine growth restriction -- 21. Preterm labor and birth / Robin G. Jordan: Social and racial disparities; Physiology of preterm birth; Complications related to prematurity; Risk factors for preterm birth; Predicting preterm birth; Diagnosing preterm birth; Management of women with preterm labor; Preterm birth prevention; Progesterone therapy; Cerclage -- 22. Hypertensive disorders in pregnancy / Robin G. Jordan: Classification of hypertensive disorders of pregnancy; Chronic hypertension; Gestational hypertension; Preeclampsia-eclampsia; Preeclampsia superimposed on chronic hypertension; Preeclampsia; HELLP syndrome; Atypical presentation preeclampsia; Prediction of preeclampsia; Prevention of preeclampsia; Long-term sequelae of preeclampsia; Risk management issues in the office setting; Interprofessional practice issues -- 23. Gestational diabetes / Kimberly K. Trout: Pathophysiology and potential problems of gestational diabetes; Prenatal screening and diagnosis of GDM; Management of gestational diabetes; Oral medications for GDM; Insulin therapy; Fetal surveillance and timing of birth; Postpartum follow-up; Scope of practice issues; Perspective on GDM risk -- 24. Other complications in pregnancy: multiple gestation, post-term pregnancy, hyperemesis, and abdominal pain / Tonya B. Nicholson: Abdominal pain in pregnancy; Hyperemesis gravidarum (HG); Multifetal pregnancy; Post-term pregnancy -- 25. Perinatal loss and grief / Robin G. Jordan: Stillbirth; Breaking the news; Care and management of women with stillbirth; Grieving and emotional care after perinatal loss; Physical care after stillbirth; Follow-up; Interconception and subsequent pregnancy care -- pt. IV. Postnatal care. 26. Physiological alterations during the postnatal period / Kimberly A. Couch and Karen DeCocker-Geist: Uterus; Lochia; Cervix; Vagina; Labia and perineum; Additional maternal alterations during the postpartum period -- 27. Components of postnatal care / Tia P. Andrighetti and Deborah Brandt Karsnitz: Assessment of maternal physical and emotional adjustment; Activity/exercise; Diet and nutrition; Lochia; Afterbirth pain; Perineal discomfort; Diureseis/diaphoresis; Constipation/hemorrhoids; Sexuality; Resumption of menses and ovulation; Contraception; Postpartum physical examination; Postpartum depression and domestic violence screening; Postnatal warning signs; Cultural considerations; Health disparities and vulnerable populations; Scope of practice considerations; Legal issues -- 28. Common complications during the postnatal period / Deborah Brandt Karsnitz:

Postpartum morbidity and mortality; Postpartum cultural considerations; Postpartum disorders -- 29. Contraception / Patricia Aikins Murphy and Leah N. Torres: Postpartum care and return to fertility after childbirth; Considerations in selecting a postpartum contraceptive method; Contraceptive methods; Tier one methods; Tier two methods; Tier three methods; Emergency contraception -- 30. Lactation and breastfeeding / Marsha Walker: Breastfeeding as a public health issue; The unique properties of human milk; Nutritional properties of human milk; Maternal and infant anatomy and physiology of lactation and breastfeeding; Promoting and supporting breastfeeding; The basics of breastfeeding support and assessment; Milk production; Breastfeeding patterns; Assessing intake; Care of the breastfeeding mother -- 31. Common breastfeeding problems / Marsha Walker: Common infant-related breastfeeding problems; Common maternal breastfeeding problems; Breast engorgement; Mastitis; Abscess; Low milk supply -- pt. V. Management of common health problems during the prenatal and postnatal periods. 32. Respiratory disorders / Janyce Cagan Agruss: Respiratory physiology and pregnancy; Asthma; Influenza; Upper respiratory infection; Pneumonia -- 33. Hematological and thromboembolic disorders / Julie A. Marfell: Anemia; Iron-deficiency anemia; Hemoglobinopathies; Folate deficiency; Vitamin B&#27;b12&#27;s deficiency; Unexplained maternal anemia; Bleeding disorders; Coagulopathies during pregnancy -- 34. Urinary tract disorders / Rhonda Arthur and Nancy Pesta Walsh: Urinary tract infection; Evaluation; Care of women with urinary tract infections; Recurrent UTI; Care of women with suspected acute pyelonephritis; Nephrolithiasis -- 35. Gastrointestinal disorders / Audra C. Malone and Karen DeCocker-Geist: Gastroenteritis; Intraheptic cholestasis of pregnancy; Cholecystitis; Appendicitis -- 36. Obesity / Cecelia M. Jevitt: Overview; Prevalence; Health disparities and cultural considerations; Personal and family considerations; Obesity physiology; Potential problems associated with obesity in childbearing women; Management of pregestational obesity; Management principles; Nutrition; Weight loss concerns; Physical activity; Comfort measures; Bariatric surgery; Scope of practice considerations; Legal and liability issues; Intrapartum and postpartum issues -- 37. Endocrine disorders / Elizabeth Gabzdyl: Thyroid disorders in pregnancy; Diagnosing thyroid disorders; Overt hypothyroidism; Subclinical hypothyroidism; Screening for hypothyroidism in pregnancy; Preconception care of a woman with hypothyroidism; Hyperthyroidism; Subclinical hyperthyroidism; Thyroid storm; Postpartum thyroiditis; Pregestational diabetes -- 38. Neurological disorders / Tonya B. Nicholson: Care of the pregnant woman; Care of pregnant women with headacle; Care of pregnant women with multiple sclerosis -- 39. Dermatological disorders / Gwendolyn Short and Elizabeth Powell Holcomb: Atopic dermatitis; Prurigo of pregnancy; Pruritic urticarial papules and plaques of pregnancy; Pruritic folliculitis of pregnancy; Pemphigoid gestationis; Impetigo herpetiformis; Intrahcpatic cholestasis of pregnancy -- 40. Infectious diseases / Jacquelyne Brooks and Elizabeth A. Parr: Cytomegalovirus; Group B streptococcus; Hepatitis infections; Parvovirus B19; Rubella; Toxoplasmosis; Varicella -- 41. Sexually transmitted infections and common vaginitis / Meghan Garland and Barbara P. Brennan: Sexually transmitted bacterial infections; Sexually transmitted viral infections; Fungal infection; Sexually transmitted parasitic infection; Sexually transmitted bacterial infection; Partner treatment of an STI; Legal requirements for reporting STI diagnosis; Psychosocial impacts of STI diagnosis -- 42. Psychological disorders / Heather Shlosser: Overview; Depression during pregnancy; Bipolar disorder in pregnancy; Generalized anxiety disorder (GAD); Scope of practice considerations.

Subjects Neonatal nursing.
Neonatal Nursing.
Patient-Centered Care.
Pregnancy--physiology.
Pregnancy Complications--nursing.
Women's Health.

Notes Includes bibliographical references and index.

Schein's common sense emergency abdominal surgery: an unconventional book for trainees and thinking surgeons

LCCN 2009921989

Type of material Book

Main title	Schein's common sense emergency abdominal surgery: an unconventional book for trainees and thinking surgeons / Moshe Schein, Paul N. Rogers, Ahmad Assalia (editors).
Edition	3rd ed.
Published/Created	Heidelberg: Springer, c2010.
Description	xxiii, 631 p.: ill.; 24 cm.
ISBN	9783540748212 3540748210
LC classification	RD540 .S335 2010
Portion of title	Common sense emergency abdominal surgery
Related names	Schein, Moshe. Rogers, Paul N. Assalia, Ahmad.
Contents	General philosophy -- The acute abdomen -- Rational diagnostic procedures -- Abdominal imaging -- Optimizing the patient -- Preoperative antibiotics -- Family, ethics, informed consent and medicolegal issues -- Before the flight: pre-op checklist -- A brief history of emergency abdominal surgery -- The incision -- Abdominal exploration: finding what is wrong -- Peritonitis: contamination and infection: principles of treatment -- The intestinal anastomosis -- Intestinal stomas -- Esophageal emergencies -- Diaphragmatic emergencies -- Upper gastrointestinal hemorrhage (and portal hypertension) -- Perforated peptic ulcer -- Acute pancreatitis -- Gallbladder and biliary emergencies Small bowel obstruction -- Acute abdominal wall hernias -- Acute mesenteric ischemia -- Inflammatory bowel disease and other types of colitis -- Colonic obstruction -- Acute diverticulitis -- Massive lower gastrointestinal

bleeding -- Acute appendicitis -- Anorectal emergencies -- Surgical complications of endoscopy -- Complications of bariatric surgery -- Complications of peritoneal dialysis -- Gynecological emergencies -- Urological emergencies -- Abdominal emergencies in infancy and childhood -- The AIDS patient -- Abdominal emergencies in the "Third World" -- Penetrating abdominal trauma -- Blunt trauma and Rx of specific injuries -- The abdominal compartment syndrome Abdominal aortic emergencies -- Abdominal drainage -- Abdominal closure -- Before landing -- Postoperative care -- Nutrition -- Postoperative antibiotics -- Postoperative ileus verus intestinal obstruction -- Intra-abdominal abscesses -- Anastomotic leaks and fistulas -- Leaks following colonic or rectal anastomoses -- Re-laparotomies and laparostomy for infection -- Abdominal wall dehiscence -- LIRS, SIRS, sepsis, MODs and tertiary peritonitis -- Wound management -- Postoperative bleeding -- The role of laparoscopy -- Complications of laparoscopic surgery -- In the aftermath and the M&M meeting.

Subjects Digestive System Diseases--surgery.
Abdomen--surgery.
Digestive System Surgical Procedures--methods.
Emergencies.
Perioperative Care--methods.
Surgical emergencies.

Notes Includes bibliographical references and index.

Surgery on the move

LCCN 2012276436

Type of material	Book
Personal name	Morgan, Jenna, author.
Main title	Surgery on the move / by Jenna Morgan, Harriet Walker, Andrew Viggars.
Published/Produced	Boca Raton, Florida CRC Press, 2013 ©2014
Description	xv, 347 pages: colour illustrations; 22 cm.
ISBN	9781444176018 (pbk) 1444176013 (pbk) 9781482208610 (ePub ebook) 148220861X (ePub ebook) 1482208628 (ebook) 9781482208627 (ebook)
Related names	Walker, Harriet, author. Viggars, Andrew, author.
Contents	14.Breast -- 14.1.Breast EMQs -- 14.2.Breast EMQ answers -- 14.3.Breast SBAs -- 14.4.Breast SBA answers -- 15.Endocrine -- 15.1.Endocrine EMQs -- 15.2.Endocrine EMQ answers -- 15.3.Endocrine SBAs -- 15.4.Endocrine SBA answers -- 16.Hepatobiliary -- 16.1.Hepatobiliary EMQs -- 16.2.Hepatobiliary EMQ answers -- 16.3.Hepatobiliary SBAs -- 16.4.Hepatobiliary SBA answers -- 17.Upper GI -- 17.1.Upper GI EMQs -- 17.2.Upper GI EMQ answers -- 17.3.Upper GI SBAs -- 17.4.Upper GI SBA answers -- 18.Colorectal -- 18.1.Colorectal EMQs -- 18.2.Colorectal EMQ answers -- 18.3.Colorectal SBAs -- 18.4.Colorectal SBA answers -- 19.Vascular -- 19.1.Vascular EMQs -- 19.2.Vascular EMQ answers -- 19.3.Vascular SBAs -- 19.4.Vascular SBA answers -- 20.Urology -- 20.1.Urology EMQs -- 20.2.Urology EMQ answers -- 20.3.Urology

SBAs -- 20.4.Urology SBA answers -- 21.Trauma and burns -- 21.1.Trauma and burns EMQs -- 21.2.Trauma and burns EMQ answers -- 21.3.Trauma and burns SBAs -- 21.4.Trauma and burns SBA answers -- 22.Post-operative care -- 22.1.Post-operative care EMQs -- 22.2.Post-operative care EMQ answers -- 22.3.Post-operative care SBAs -- 22.4.Post-operative care SBA answers.

Subjects	Surgery.
Notes	Includes index.
Series	Medicine on the move

The 5-minute pediatric consult

LCCN	2012012664
Type of material	Book
Main title	The 5-minute pediatric consult / editor, M. William Schwartz; associate editors, Louis M. Bell, Jr. ... [et al.]; assistant editor, Charles I. Schwartz.
Edition	6th ed.
Published/Created	Philadelphia: Wolters Kluwer/Lippincott Williams & Wilkins, c2012.
Description	xxx, 1113 p.: ill.; 28 cm.
ISBN	9781451116564 (hardback: alk. paper) 145111656X (hardback: alk. paper)
LC classification	RJ48 .A15 2012
Variant title	Five-minute pediatric consult
Related names	Schwartz, M. William, 1935-
Summary	"The 5 Minute Pediatric Consult provides immediate, practical advice on problems seen in infants, children, and adolescents. More than 450 diseases and conditions are covered in the fast-access two-page outline format that makes The 5-

Minute Consult Series titles so popular among busy clinicians. Other features include a Chief Complaints section addressing the workup and treatment of 50 signs and symptoms, plus a medication index, syndromes glossary, surgical glossary, laboratory values, and tables all for quick reference saving you time and helping to treat your patients more efficiently. In this sixth edition, the 5 Minute Pediatric Consult also offers free 30 day access to the 5minuteconsult Pediatric website -- a clinical decision support tool -- that can be accessed by the health care providers to address questions on-the-go via website or mobile. New Features: New topics for this edition include: Amenorrhea, Asberger Syndrome, Dental Trauma, Head banging, Mental Retardation, Narcolepsy, Obsessive Compulsive Disorder, Separation Anxiety and Social Anxiety Free 30 Day Access to the 5minuteconsult Pediatric Website Includes More than 450 diseases and conditions to support your patient care decisions Patient education handouts from AAP to help educate your patients Hundreds of Images from Chung's "Visual Diagnosis and Treatment in Pediatrics" and other reputable sources to provide you with quick visual guidance Immunization schedules and charts at your fingertips to save you time from searching Content is optimized for handheld devices so you have access to the content anytime, anywhere Updates to content made on a regular basis to keep you abreast of the latest content Visit 5minuteconsult.com and click on the "go to pediatric consult tab" to learn more about your free access and begin using today!"-- Provided by publisher.

Contents Abdominal Mass -- Abdominal migraine -- Abdominal pain -- Abnormal bleeding -- Acetaminophen poisoning -- Acne -- Acquired hypothyroidism -- Acute drug withdrawal -- Acute kidney injury -- Acute lymphoblastic leukemia -- Acute myeloid leukemia -- Adenovirus infection -- Alcohol (ethanol) intoxication -- Allergic child -- Alopecia (hair loss) -- Alpha-1-Antitrypsin defficiency -- Altitude illness -- Amblyopia -- Amebiasis -- Amenorrhea -- Anearobic infections -- Anaphylaxis -- Anemia of chronic disease (Anemia of inflammation) -- Anicryptococcal infections -- Ankylosing spondylitis -- Anomalous coronary artery -- Anorexia nervosa -- Anthrax -- Aplastic anemia -- Appendicitis -- Arthritis, Juvenile idiopathic (Rheumatoid) -- Ascaris lumbricoides -- Ascites -- Aspergillosis -- Asplenia/Hyposplenia -- Asthma -- Ataxia -- Atelectasis -- Atopic dermatitis -- Atrial septal defect -- Attention-Deficit/Hyperactivity disorder (ADHD) -- Atypical Mycobacterial infections -- Autism/Pervasive developmental disorder (PDD) Spectrum -- Autoimmune hemolytic anemia -- Avascular (aseptic) necrosis of the femoral head (HIP) -- Babesiosis -- Back pain -- Barotitis -- Bell palsy -- Bezoars -- Biliary Atresia -- Blastomycosis -- Blepharitis -- Bone marrow and stem cell transplant -- Botulism -- Brain abscess -- Brain injury, Traumatic -- Brain tumor -- Branchial cleft malformations -- Breast Abscess -- Breastfeeding -- Breastfeeding Jaundice and breast milk jaundice -- Breath-holding spells -- Bronchiolitis (See also: Respiratory syncytial virus) -- Bronchopulmonary dysplasia (Chronic lung disease of prematurity) -- Bruising -- Bruxism -- Bulimia -- C 1 Esterase inhibitor deficiency -- Campylobacter infections -- Candidiasis -- Carbon monoxide poisoning -- Cardimyopathy -- Cataract -- Cat-scratch disease -- Cavernous Sinus Syndrome -- Cavernous transformation and portal vein obstruction -- Celiac disease -- Cellulitis -- Cerebral palsy -- Cervicitis -- Chancroid -- Chest Pain – Chickenpox(Varicella, Herpes Zoster) -- Child abuse, Physical -- Chlamydial infections -- Cholelithiasis -- Cholera -- Chronic Diarrhea -- Chronic granulmatous disease -- Chronic hepatitis -- Chronic kidney disease -- Cirrhosis -- Cleft lip and palate -- Clubfoot -- Coarctation of aorta -- Coccidioidomycosis -- Colic -- Coma -- Common variable immunodeficiency -- Complement deficiency -- Concussion -- Congenital hepatic fibrosis -- Congenital hypothyroidism -- Congestive heart failure -- Conjunctivitis -- Constipation -- Contact Dermatitis -- Contraception -- Cor pulmonale -- Costochondritis -- Cough -- Crohn disease -- Croup -- Crying -- Cryptococcal infections -- Cryptorchidism -- Cryptosporidiosis -- Cushing Syndrome (Adrenal Excess) -- Cutaneous Larva Migrans -- Cyclospora -- Cystic fibrosis -- Cytomegalovirus infection -- 22q11.2 Deletion Syndrome (Digeorge Syndrome) -- Dental/Oral Pain and urgencies -- Dermatomyositis/ Polymyositis -- Developmental disabilities --

Developmental dysplasia of the hip -- Diabetes insipidus -- Diabetes mellitus -- Diabetic ketoacidosis Diaper rash -- Diaphragmatic hernia (Congenital) -- Diarrhea -- Diphtheria -- Diskitis -- Disorders of sex development -- Disseminated intravascular coagulation -- Down (Trisomy 21) Syndrome -- Drowning -- Dysfunctional uterine bleeding -- Dysmenorrhea -- Dyspnea -- Dysuria -- Earache -- Edema -- Ehrlichiosis and anaplasmosis -- Encephalitis -- Encopresis -- Endocarditis -- Enuresis -- Endocarditis -- Epiglottitis -- Epstein Barr virus (Infectious Mononucleosis -- Erythema multiforme -- Erythema Nodosum -- Ewing Sarcoma -- Exstrophy of the bladder, cloacal exstrophy, and epispadias -- Failure to thrive -- Feeding disorders -- Fetal alcohol syndrome -- Fever and petechiae -- Fever of unknown cause -- Floppy infant syndrome -- Food allergy -- Food poisoning or foodborne illness -- Fragile X syndrome -- Frostbite -- Functional diarrhea of infancy or toddler's diarrhea -- Fungal skin infections (Dermatophyte infections, Candidiasis, and Tinea Versicolor) -- Gastritis -- Gastroesophageal reflux -- German measles (third disease, Rubella) -- Giardiasis -- Gingivitis -- Glaucoma--congenital -- Glomerulonephritis -- Gluecose-6-phosphate dehydrogenase deficiency -- Goiter -- Gonococcal infections -- Graft versus host disease -- Graves disease -- Growth hormone deficiency -- Guillain-Barre syndrome -- Gynecomastia -- Hand, foot, and mouth disease -- Hantavirus -- Head banging -- Headache and migraine -- Heat stroke and related illness --

Hemangiomas and other vascular lesions -- Hematuria -- Hemolysis -- Hemolysis -- Hemolytic disease of the newborn -- Hemolytic uremic syndrome -- Hemophilia -- Hemoptysis -- Henoch-Schonlein purpura -- Hepatic failure -- Hepatomegaly -- Hereditary Angioedema -- Hereditary spherocytosis -- Heroin intoxication -- Herpes simplex virus -- Hiccups -- Hirschsprung disease -- Histiocytosis -- Histoplasmosis -- Hodgkin Lymphoma -- Human immunodeficiency virus infection -- Human papilloma virus -- Hydrocephalus -- Hydronephrosis -- Hyperimmunoglobulinemia E Syndrome -- Hyperinsulinism -- Hyperlipidemia -- Hypertention -- Hypogrammaglobulinemia -- Hypoparathyroidism -- Hypoplastic left heart syndrome -- Hypospadias -- Idiopathic intracranial hypertension (Pseudotumor cerebri) -- Idiopathic Thrombocytopenic purpura -- Immune deficiency -- Immunoglobulin a deficiency -- Imperforate anus -- Impetigo -- In Inappropriate antidiuretic hormone secretion -- Infantile spasms -- Influenza -- Inguinal hernia -- Intestinal obstruction -- Intoeing-tibial torsion -- Intracranial hemorrhage -- Intussusception -- Iron deficiency anemia -- Iron poisoning -- Irritable bowel syndrome -- Jaundice -- Kawasaki disease -- Knee pain, Anterior/Patellofemoral malalignment syndrome -- Lacrimal duct obstruction -- Lactos intolerance -- Lead poisoning -- Learning disabilities -- Luekocytosis -- Lice (Pediculosis) -- Lower GI bleeding -- Lupus erythematosus -- Lyme disease -- Lymphadenopathy -- Malabsorption -- Malaria --

Mammalian bites -- Mastoiditis -- Measles (Rubeola, first disease) -- Meckel diverticulum -- Mediastinal mass -- Megaloblastic ancmia -- Meningitis -- Meningococcemia -- Mental retardation -- Mesenteric adenitis -- Metabolic diseases in hypoglycemic newborns -- Metabolic diseases in acidotic newborns -- Metabolic diseases in Hyperammonemic newborns -- Metabolic syndrome -- Methemoglobinemia -- Microcytic anemia -- Milia -- Milk protein intolerance -- Mumps/Parotitis -- Munchausen syndrome by proxy -- Muscular dystrophies -- Myasthenia gravis -- Myocarditis -- Narcolepsy -- Neck masses -- Necrotizing entercolitis -- Neonatal alloimmune thrombocytopenia -- Neonatal apnea -- Neonatal cholestasis -- Nephrotic syndrome -- Neural tube defects -- Neuroblastoma -- Neurofibromatosis -- Neutropenia -- Non-Hodgkin Lymphoma -- Nosebleeds (Epistaxis) -- Obesity -- Obsessive compulsive disorder -- Obstetric brachial plexus (ERB) palsy -- Omphalitis -- Osteogenesis imperfecta -- Osteosarcoma -- Osteomyelitis -- Otitis externa -- Otitis media -- Pallor -- Pancreatic Pseudocyst -- Pancreatitis -- Panhypopituitarism -- Parvovirus B 19 (Erythema Infectiosum, fifth disease) -- Patent ductus arteriosus -- Pelvic inflammatory disease (PID) -- Penile and foreskin problems -- Pericarditis -- Periodic breathing -- Periorbital cellulitis -- Perirectal abscess -- Peritonitis -- Peritonsillar abscess -- Persistent Pulmonary Hypertension of the newborn (PPHN) -- Perthes disease -- Pertussis -- Pharyngitis -- Photosensitivity --

Pinworms -- Plague -- Pleural effusion -- Pneumoystic Jiroveci (Previously known as Pneumocystic Carnii Pneumonis) -- Pneumonia--Bacterial -- Pneumothorax -- Polyarteritis Nodosa -- Polycystic kidney disease -- Polycystic ovary syndrome -- Polycythemia -- Polyps, intestinal -- Porencephaly cortical dysplasia/neuronal migration disorders-malformations of cortical development -- Portal hypertension -- Posterior urethral valve -- Premature adrenarche -- Premature thelarche -- Premenstrual syndrome (PMS) -- Primary adrenal insufficiency -- Prion diseases (Transmissible spongiform encephalophathies) -- Probiotics -- Prolonged QT interval syndrome -- Protein-Energy malnutrition (Kwashiorkor) -- Proteinuria -- Prune belly syndrome -- Pruritus -- Psittacosis -- Psoriasis -- Pubertal delay -- Pulmonary embolism -- Pulmonary hypertension -- Purpura fulminans -- Pyelonephritis -- Pyloric stenosis -- Rabies -- Rectal prolapse -- Refractive error -- Renal artery stenosis -- Renal tubular acidosis -- Renal venous thrombosis -- Respiratory syncytial virus (RSV) -- Retinoblastoma -- Retropharyngeal abscess -- Reye Syndrome -- Rhabdomyolysis -- Rhabdomyosarcoma -- Rheumatic fever -- Rhinitis, Allergic -- Rickets -- Rickettsial disease -- Rocky Mountain Spotted Fever -- Roseola -- Rotavirus -- Salicylate poisoning (Aspirin) -- Salmonella infections -- Sarcoidosis -- Scabies -- Scarlet fever -- Scleroderma -- Scoliosis (Idiopathic) -- Seborrheic dermatitis -- Seizures-febrile -- Seizures, partial and generalized -- Separation anxiety disorder -- Sepsis -- Septic arthritis -- Serum Sickness -- Severe acute respiratory syndrome (SARS) -- Severe combined immunodeficiency -- Sexual abuse -- Sexual ambiguity -- Sexual precocity -- Short-bowel syndrome -- Short stature -- Sickle cell disease -- Sinusitis -- Sleep apnea--obstructive sleep apnea syndrome -- Slipped capital femoral epiphysis -- Smallpox (Variola virus) -- Snake and insect bites -- Social anxiety disorder -- Sore throat -- Speech delay -- Speech problems -- Spinal muscular atrophy -- Splenomegaly -- Staphylococcal scaled skin syndrome (SSSS) -- Status epilepticus -- Stevens-Johnson syndrome and toxic epidermal necrolysis -- Stomatitis -- Strabismus -- Strep infection: invasive Group A Ç-hemolytic streptococcus -- Stroke -- Stuttering -- Subdural hematoma -- Substance use disorders -- Sudden Infant Death Syndrome (SIDS) -- Suicide -- Superior Mesenteric Artery syndrome -- Superior Mesenteric artery syndrome -- Supraventricular tachycardia -- Sympathomimetic poisoning -- Syncope -- Synovitis--transient -- Syphilis -- Tapeworm -- Teething -- Tendonitis -- Teratoma -- Tenanus -- Tetralogy of Fallot -- Thalassemia -- Thoracic insufficiency syndrome -- Thrombosis -- Tick fever -- Tics -- Toxic alcohols -- Toxic Shock syndrome -- Toxoplasmosis -- Tracheitis -- Tracheoesophageal fistula and esophageal atresia -- Tracheomalacia/laryngomalacia -- Transfusion reaction -- Transient erythroblastopenia of childhood -- Transient Trachypnea of the Newborn (TTN) -- Transposition of the great arteries -- Transverse myelitis -- Trichinosis -- Tuberculosis -- Tuberous

	sclerosis complex -- Tularemia -- Ulcerative colitis -- Upper gastrointestional bleeding -- Ureteropelvic junction obstruction -- Urethral prolapse -- Urinary tract infection -- Urticaria -- Vaccine adverse events -- Vaginitis -- Vascular brain lesions (Congenial) -- Ventricular septal defect -- Ventricular tachycardia -- Vesicoureteral reflux -- Viral hepatitis -- Volvulus -- Vomiting -- Von Willebrand disease -- Warts -- Weight loss -- West Nile Virus (And other Arbovirus Encephalitis) -- Wheezing -- Wilms tumor -- Wilson disease -- Wiskott-Aldrich syndrome -- Yersinia enterocolitica.
Subjects	Pediatrics--Handbooks, manuals, etc.
	Pediatrics.
	Pediatrics--Handbooks.
Notes	Includes bibliographical references and index.
Series	5-minute consult series
	5-minute consult.

The complete vegetarian: the essential guide to good health

LCCN	2007030754
Type of material	Book
Main title	The complete vegetarian: the essential guide to good health / edited by Peggy Carlson.
Published/Created	Urbana: University of Illinois Press, c2009.
Description	xii, 361 p.: ill.; 26 cm.
Links	Table of contents only http://www.loc.gov/catdir/toc/ecip0723/2007030754.html
ISBN	9780252032516 (cloth: alk. paper)
	0252032519 (cloth: alk. paper)
	9780252075063 (pbk.: alk. paper)
	0252075064 (pbk.: alk. paper)
LC classification	TX392 .C69 2009

Related names Carlson, Peggy.

Contents Introduction / Peggy Carlson -- Protein / Virginia Messina -- Fats / Brenda Davis -- Fiber / Peggy Carlson -- Iron / Dina Aronson -- Calcium and vitamin D / Suzanne Havala Hobbs, John J.B. Anderson -- Vitamin B12 / Michael A. Klaper -- Zinc / Virginia Messina, Reed Mangels -- Other vitamins and minerals / Reed Mangels -- Heart disease / Peggy Carlson -- Cancer / Peggy Carlson -- Hypertension / James Craner -- Stroke / Peggy Carlson -- Obesity and a vegetarian diet / Sudha Raj Diabetes and vegetarian diets / Peggy Carlson -- Osteoporosis / John J.B. Anderson, Suzanne Havala Hobbs -- Gallbladder disease, diverticulitis, appendicitis, kidney stones, and kidney failure / Valerie Kurtzhalls, Peggy Carlson -- Vegetarian diets and children / Jeanene Fogli, Carol M. Meerschaert -- Pregnancy and lactation / Reed Mangels -- Optimal nutrition for active vegetarians and vegetarian athletes / D. Enette Larson-Meyer, Mary Helen Niemeyer -- Environmental and food safety aspects of vegetarian diets / Carl V. Phillips, Simon K. Emms, Erin L. Kraker -- Planning nutritious vegetarian diets / Cheryl Sullivan -- Conclusion: summary of protective factors / Virginia Messina, Peggy Carlson.

Subjects Vegetarianism--Popular works.
Nutrition--Popular works.
Diet, Vegetarian--Popular Works.
Chronic Disease--prevention & control--Popular Works.
Micronutrients--Popular Works.
Nutritional Requirements--Popular Works.

Notes	Includes bibliographical references and index.
Series	The food series Food series.

Ultrasound for surgeons

LCCN	2003025277
Type of material	Book
Personal name	Frankel, Heidi L.
Main title	Ultrasound for surgeons / Heidi L. Frankel.
Published/Created	Georgetown, Tex., U.S.A.: Landes Bioscience, c2005.
Description	172 p.: ill.; 21 cm.
Links	Table of contents http://www.loc.gov/catdir/toc/ecip0411/2003025277.html
ISBN	1570595976
LC classification	RD33.7 .F73 2005
Contents	Education credentialing and getting started / Vincente Gracias, Heidi Frankel and Ronald Gross -- FAST (focused assessment by sonography in trauma) / Ronald Gross -- Chest trauma / Frank Davis and M. Gage Ochsner -- Abdominal aortic aneurysm screening / David Pilcher -- Pediatric applications / Oluyinka Olutoye, Richard Bellah and Perry Stafford -- Appendicitis / S.C. Chen -- Surveillance of deep vein thrombosis (DVT) / Rajan Gupta and Jeffrey Carpenter -- Insertion of central catheters / Tarek Razek and Michael Russell -- Transcranial Doppler / George Counelis and Grant Sinson -- Diagnosis and treatment of fluid collections and other pathology / Mark McKenney and S. Morad Hameed -- Use in the operating room / P.V. Gallagher, David Wherry and Richard Charnley -- Use in the operating room--laparoscopic / Rajesh

	Gandhi -- Breast ultrasound / Sheryl Gabram and Nicos Labropoulos -- Vascular / David Neschis and Jeffrey Carpenter -- Rectal / John Winston and Lee Smith.
Subjects	Ultrasonics in surgery. Operative ultrasonography. Ultrasonography--methods--Handbooks. Surgical Procedures, Operative--methods--Handbooks.
Notes	Includes bibliographical references and index.
Series	Vademecum

Williams manual of pregnancy complications

LCCN	2012026521
Type of material	Book
Main title	Williams manual of pregnancy complications / senior editor, Kenneth J. Leveno; associate editors, James M. Alexander ... [et al.].
Edition	23rd ed.
Published/Created	New York: McGraw-Hill Professional, c2013.
ISBN	9780071765626 (alk. paper)
Variant title	Manual of pregnancy compilations
Related titles	William's manual of obstetrics. Williams obstetrics.
Related names	Leveno, Kenneth J. Alexander, James M., 1965-
Summary	"The only pocket manual derived from Williams Obstetrics, 23e -- completely updated and now in full color Williams Manual of Pregnancy Complications, 23e is a carry-anywhere, condensed guide to the Williams protocols for diagnosis and management of complications and illnesses during pregnancy. Reflecting the rigorously referenced, evidence-based approach

of the parent text, the manual delivers essential information on: Prenatal screening Mediation use in pregnancy Hypertension disorders in pregnancy Pain management dosages Procedures for complicated labor and delivery, hemoglobinopathies, and more Thoroughly cross-referenced to Williams Obstetrics, 23e for the latest literature citations, this edition is enhanced by a new full-color presentation, more tables and algorithms, and an increased emphasis on diagnosis and treatment. There is no faster or more efficient way to access the key facts, diagnostic tools, and treatment guidelines found in Williams Obstetrics, 23e than this authoritative, streamlined sourcebook"--Provided by publisher.

Contents Machine generated contents note: Part I: Obstetrical Complications due to Pregnancy 1. Early Pregnancy Loss 2. Ectopic Pregnancy 3. Screening for Neural-Tube Defects, Down Syndrome, and Heritable Genetic Diseases 4. Prenatal Diagnosis 5. Chromosomal Abnormalities 6. Single-Gene (Mendelian) Disorders 7. Nonmendelian Disorders 8. Teratology, Medications, and Substance Abuse 9. Ultrasound Imaging Including Doppler Velocimetry 10. Oligohydramnios 11. Hydramnios 12. Antepartum Fetal Testing 13. Intrapartum Fetal Heart Rate Assessment 14. Abnormal Labor and Delivery 15. Chorioamnionitis 16. Shoulder Dystocia 17. Breech Delivery 18. Prior Cesarean Delivery 19. Uterine Rupture 20. Hysterectomy Following Delivery 21. Postpartum and Postoperative Infections 22. Septic Pelvic Thrombophlebitis 23.

Gestational Hypertension and Preeclampsia 24. Eclampsia 25. Placental Abruption 26. Placenta Previa 27. Fetal-to-Maternal Hemorrhage 28. Hemorrhage Immediately Following Delivery 29. Transfusion of Blood Products for Obstetrical Hemorrhage 30. Amnionic Fluid Embolism 31. Fetal Death and Delayed Delivery 32. Preterm Birth: Definitions, Consequences, and Causes 33. Prediction of Preterm Birth 34. Preterm Ruptured Membranes 35. Preterm Birth: Intact Membranes 36. Incompetent Cervix 37. Postterm Pregnancy 38. Fetal Growth Restriction 39. Macrosomia 40. Twin Pregnancy: Overview 41. Complications Unique to Twins 42. Triplets and More 43. Selective Reduction or Termination of Multifetal Pregnancy 44. Gestational Trophoblastic Disease Part II: Medical and Surgical Complications during Pregnancy 45. Active Pulmonary Edema and Adult Respiratory Distress Syndrome 46. Pulmonary Artery Catheterization 47. Chronic Hypertension 48. Heart Disease in Pregnancy 49. Pneumonia 50. Asthma 51. Tuberculosis, Sarcoid and Cystic Fibrosis 52. Thromboembolic Disease 53. Thrombophilias 54. Antiphospholipid Antibody Syndrome 55. Systemic Lupus Erythematosus 56. Rheumatoid Arthritis and Other Connective-Tissue Disorders 57. Hyperemesis Gravidarum 58. Cholestasis of Pregnancy 59. Diseases of the Gallbladder and Pancreas 60. Appendicitis 61. Viral Hepatitis 62. Acute Fatty Liver of Pregnancy 63. Asymptomatic Bacteriuria (ASB) 64. Cystitis 65. Acute Pyelonephritis 66. Nephrolithiasis 67. Acute and Chronic Renal Failure 68. Anemia 69.

Hemoglobinopathies 70. Thrombocytopenia 71. Gestational Diabetes 72. Pregestational Overt Diabetes 73. Hypothyroidism 74. Hyperthyroidism 75. Postpartum Thyroiditis 76. Epilepsy 77. Cerebrovascular Diseases 78. Other Neurologic Disorders 79. Psychiatric Illnesses During Pregnancy 80. Postpartum Depression 81. Cancer During Pregnancy 82. Dermatological Disorders 83. Sexually Transmitted Diseases 84. Group A and B Streptococcus Infections 85. Human Immunodeficiency Virus 86. Cytomegalovirus, Parvovirus, Varicella, Rubella, Toxoplasmosis, Listeria, and Malaria 87. Trauma in Pregnancy 88. Surgery During Pregnancy Part III: Complications in the Fetus or Newborn Infant 89. Resuscitation of the Newborn Infant 90. Neonatal Complications of Prematurity 91. Rh Disease and Other Isoimmunization 92. Injuries to the Fetus and Newborn 93. Meconium Aspiration, Cerebral Palsy, and Other Diseases of the Fetus and Newborn 94. Stillbirth Appendix A: Diagnostic Indices in Pregnancy Appendix B: Ultrasound Reference Tables Appendix C: Radiation Dosimetry Appendix D: Umbilical Cord Blood Gas Analysis Index.

Subjects Pregnancy Complications--Handbooks.

Notes Rev. ed. of: William's manual of obstetrics / Kenneth J. Leveno ... [et al.]. 22nd ed. c2007.
Derived from: Williams obstetrics. 23rd ed. / [edited by] F. Gary Cunningham ... [et al.]. c2010.
Includes bibliographical references and index.

RELATED NOVA PUBLICATIONS

APPENDICITIS: RISK FACTORS, MANAGEMENT STRATEGIES AND CLINICAL IMPLICATIONS

Angela S. Marmo (Editor)

ISBN: 978-1-63321-526-9 Publication Date 2014
Binding: Hardcover Series: Emergency and Intensive Care Medicine

Appendicitis remains one of the most common surgical emergencies, with approximately 200,000 annual cases in the United States and a lifetime risk of 8%. The treatment of appendicitis has evolved significantly, from the first reported appendectomy in 1736 at St. George's Hospital in London. This book discusses several topics on appendicitis including the surgical management of appendicitis; pediatric advanced appendicitis; acute appendicitis; treatment strategies; risk factors and clinical implications.

Chapter 21 Management of Acute Appendicitis in Pregnancy and the Puerperium
Ekundayo S. Garba, Robert B. Sanda, Department of Surgery, Ahmadu Bello University, Zaria, Nigeria

APPENDICITIS*

Henri Kotobi[1,†] and Taieb Chouikh[2,‡]

[1]Pediatric Surgery Department,
Hôpital Universitaire Armand Trousseau, Paris, France
[2]Tunis School of Medecine University El Manar, Tunisia
Department of Paediatric Surgery,
Hôpital Universitaire Necker-Enfants malades Hospital, Paris, France
Hopital Robert Ballanger, Aulnay-sous-Bois, France

Acute appendicitis (AA) remains the most common visceral paediatric surgery emergency in developed countries [1]. Since the 90s, the radiological progress allowed a considerable improvement in the diagnosis of acute paediatric appendicitis. Nevertheless, it is not always easy to have an accurate diagnosis.

Two risks persist in the management of acute paediatric appendicitis: the delay in the diagnosis and a high rate of false positive diagnosis, which justifies being interested in this entity in all points of view (epidemiological, diagnosis and therapeutic management).

---

* The full version of this chapter can be found in *Pediatric Surgery Handbook for Residents and Medical Students*, edited by Taieb Chouikh, published by Nova Science Publishers, Inc, New York, 2017.

† MD, Pediatric Surgeon.

‡ MD, Special Registrar, Formely Pediatric Surgery assistant Professor.

INDEX

A

B

C

D

E

G

H

I

K

L

M

N

O

P

Appendicitis: Risk Factors, Management Strategies and Clinical Implications

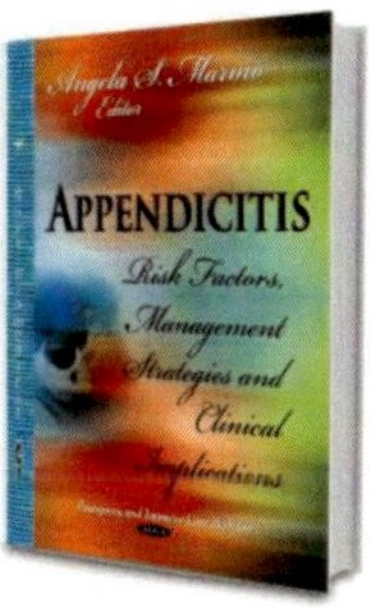

Editor: Angela S. Marmo

Series: Emergency and Intensive Care Medicine

Book Description: This book discusses several topics on appendicitis including the surgical management of appendicitis; pediatric advanced appendicitis; acute appendicitis; treatment strategies; risk factors and clinical implications.

Hardcover ISBN: 978-1-63321-526-9
Retail Price: $255

Acute Appendicitis in Pregnancy

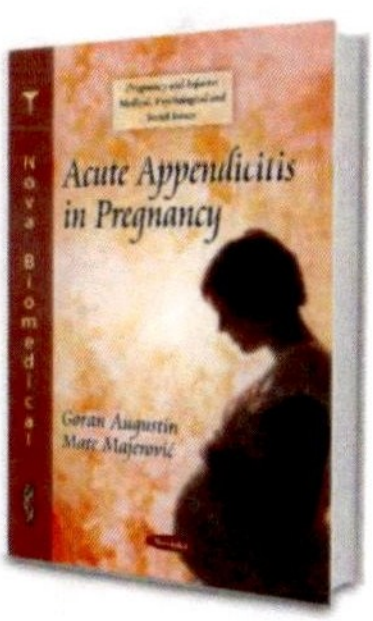

Authors: Goran Augustin, Mate Majeroviæ (University of Zagreb, Zagreb, Croatia)

Series: Pregnancy and Infants: Medical, Psychological and Social Issues

Book Description: Acute appendicitis is present in one in 500 to 2000 pregnancies (which amounts to 25% of operative indications for the acute abdomen in pregnancy). This book examines the occurrence, symptoms and severity of acute appendicitis in pregnancy.

Softcover ISBN: 978-1-61122-581-5
Retail Price: $69

Appendicitis: Symptoms, Diagnosis, and Treatments

Editor: William L. Ryan

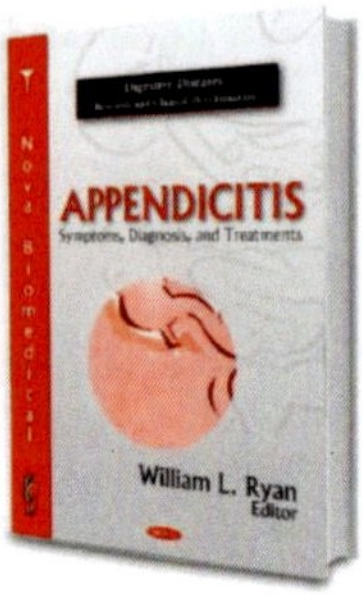

Series: Digestive Diseases - Research and Clinical Developments

Book Description: This book presents research data from across the globe in the study of appendicitis, its symptoms, diagnosis and treatments. Included herein are topics such as appendicitis during pregnancy; antibiotic therapy alone in the management of acute appendicitis; diagnostic strategies and immunology in acute appendicitis; and utilization of the Alvarado score to perform CT for acute appendicitis.

Hardcover ISBN: 978-1-61761-737-9
Retail Price: $130